T0224858

Theorising Occupational Therapy Practice in Diverse Settings

Practice theory provides a way of understanding everyday life, but until now its application in occupational therapy has not been much developed. *Theorising Occupational Therapy Practice in Diverse Settings* draws on practice theory to explore the conditions for occupational therapy practice in a variety of clinical and non-traditional settings.

With examples from around the globe, the chapters of the first section unfold practice theory perspectives of occupational therapy history, the management of occupational therapists in health systems, professional roles and working contexts. A bridging chapter reviews this development and sets out some of the global social phenomena that shaped occupational therapy; including colonialism and social inequality. The authors look forward to where the profession finds itself at present, in terms of social and health needs, power structures, occupational therapy theory and emerging areas of practice. The second section of the book considers how occupational therapists are responding to the challenges facing the profession in relation to issues of access, resources and change. A final chapter reviews how occupational therapy can meet the health-related occupational needs of individuals, communities and populations throughout the 21st century. While acknowledging the complexity of occupational, health and social needs, the book enables readers to relate occupational therapy aims and objectives effectively to pragmatic strategies for dealing with the realities of working in different settings.

With numerous case examples, this is an important new text for students and practitioners of occupational therapy. It is relevant both for those working in, or preparing for, placements in mainstream health and social care services, or in community interest companies, charities and social enterprises.

Jennifer Creek became an occupational therapist in 1970 and has worked in adult mental health, adult learning disabilities, professional education, primary care and mental health promotion. Jennifer has edited and co-edited textbooks and collections of essays on occupational therapy philosophy, theory and professional reasoning.

Nick Pollard is a senior lecturer in occupational therapy who formerly worked in severe and enduring mental health services, having completed training in 1991. He has written and presented extensively on community-based rehabilitation and critical explorations of occupational therapy.

Michael Allen is a sociologist and researcher specialising in social practice theory. He studied at the University of Hull and the University of Leeds before moving to the DEMAND Centre at Lancaster University in 2014, to take up a PhD studentship focusing on the energy demand of leisure activities.

Theorising Occupational Therapy Practice in Diverse Settings

Edited by Jennifer Creek, Nick Pollard, and Michael Allen

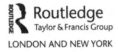

LONDON AND NEW YORK

Cover image: © Getty Images

First published 2023
by Routledge
4 Park Square, Milton Park, Abingdon, Oxon OX14 4RN

and by Routledge
605 Third Avenue, New York, NY 10158

Routledge is an imprint of the Taylor & Francis Group, an informa business

British Library Cataloguing-in-Publication Data
A catalogue record for this book is available from the British Library

Library of Congress Cataloguing-in-Publication Data
Names: Creek, Jennifer, editor.| Pollard, Nick, MSc(OT), editor. |
Allen, Michael (Sociologist), editor.
Title: Theorising occupational therapy practice in diverse settings / edited by Jennifer Creek, Nick Pollard and Michael Allen.
Description: Abingdon, Oxon ; New York, NY : Routledge, 2023. |
Includes bibliographical references and index.
Identifiers: LCCN 2022025168 (print) | LCCN 2022025169 (ebook) |
ISBN 9780367860769 (hardback) | ISBN 9780367860752 (paperback) |
ISBN 9781003016755 (ebook)
Subjects: LCSH: Occupational therapy.
Classification: LCC RM735.A6 T44 2022 (print) | LCC RM735.A6 (ebook) |
DDC 615.8/515--dc23/eng/20220804
LC record available at https://lccn.loc.gov/2022025168
LC ebook record available at https://lccn.loc.gov/2022025169

ISBN: 978-0-367-86076-9 (hbk)
ISBN: 978-0-367-86075-2 (pbk)
ISBN: 978-1-003-01675-5 (ebk)

DOI: 10.4324/9781003016755

Typeset in Times New Roman
by MPS Limited, Dehradun

In memory of Professor Averil Stewart, the UK's first professor of occupational therapy and former Head of Occupational Therapy at Queen Margaret University,

and Melanie Bryer, one of the founding lecturers at Sheffield Hallam University's occupational therapy programmes.

Contents

List of tables   ix
List of boxes   x
List of contributors   xii
Foreword   xiv
Preface   xvi
Acknowledgements   xviii

1   History and early development of occupational therapy   1
    JENNIFER CREEK AND MICHAEL ALLEN

2   Managerialism and health services   24
    JENNIFER CREEK

3   Space-time, temporality and professional roles   41
    KATE SHERRY, JENNIFER CREEK, AND MICHAEL ALLEN

4   Space-time, place and working contexts   61
    KATE SHERRY AND ANRI-LOUISE OOSTHUIZEN

5   The current position of occupational therapy theory and
    practice   78
    NICK POLLARD

6   Access   100
    ELLY BADCOCK, ELISE BROMANN BUKHAVE, AND JENNIFER CREEK

7   Resources   122
    TEMPLE MOORE AND JENNIFER CREEK

8   Change in occupational therapy   143
    ANA CARREIRA DE MELLO, TAIS QUEVEDO MARCOLINO, AND
    NICK POLLARD

9   Where we want to be   165
    NICK POLLARD AND JENNIFER CREEK

    Glossary   183
    Index   188

Tables

1.1   The occupational therapy curriculum   11
7.1   Resources for occupational therapy   123
7.2   Resources utilised by CircusAid   132

Boxes

1.1   Women's rights in the UK – 1800–1928   2
1.2   Housing reform in the United Kingdom and the United
       States – 1848–1875   3
1.3   Settlement house movement – 1884   5
1.4   The arts and crafts movement – 1880–1920   6
1.5   Pragmatism   7
2.1   Conflict of interest   31
2.2   Task competence without professional judgement   32
2.3   Following procedure   33
3.1   Aligning the values and goals of occupational therapy with the
       employing organisation   48
3.2   How healthcare funding influences time use   49
3.3   Features of a profession   50
3.4   Family decision-making: Immediate needs versus future orientation   57
4.1   A pavement as both objective and lived space   63
4.2   'Do you do massage?' Context 1   68
4.3   'Do you do massage?' Context 2   68
4.4   'Do you do massage?' Context 3   69
4.5   'Do you do massage?' Context 4   69
5.1   Occupational therapist as an advocate   79
5.2   A constellation of practice   81
5.3   Exporting occupational therapy as a new health technology   84
5.4   The unequal impact of climate change   86
5.5   Food inequity in a wealthy country   87
5.6   Social occupational therapy   94
6.1   The impact of barriers to access   102
6.2   Disability perspective   102
6.3   Barriers to access in everyday life   105
6.4   Three qualities of connective tissue in hospital life   106
6.5   Exclusion from occupational therapy services   107
6.6   How digital solutions can challenge the homeless   109
6.7   Disability and personhood   112
6.8   Naming and framing an access problem   114
6.9   Working with the client   116
6.10   Basing practice on principles   117
6.11   Temporal considerations   118

7.1 Negotiating resource allocation at the macro-level 125
7.2 Unequal opportunities for development 126
7.3 Infrastructure, devices and consumables in the kitchen 127
7.4 Training for staff working with child refugees 128
7.5 Accommodating the abilities and needs of team members 133
8.1 The elements of cooking as a practice 144
8.2 The hospital as an evolving complex of practices 145
8.3 The meaning of the car in community occupational therapy practice 147
8.4 The development of mental healthcare in Brazil 148
8.5 The Dynamic Occupational Therapy Method 151
9.1 Digital marginalisation 169
9.2 Improvisation 171
9.3 Ubuntu 172
9.4 Working independently 176

Contributors

Rafaela Arrigoni has a residency in mental health and clinical training in the Dynamic Occupational Therapy Method (DOTM). Rafaela has worked in the area of child mental health in primary care and in Psychosocial Care Centres (CAPSij). Currently, she works in private practice with adolescents and adults.

Elly Badcock is an occupational therapist in a community learning disability team. She is especially interested in how people with a learning disability experience and wield power, and has recently published research around this dynamic in health and social care settings.

Ana Paula Briguet has clinical training in the DOTM. Her areas of expertise are mental health and family health, with more than 20 years of experience in community mental health services in the Unified Health System in Brazil, as a practitioner and manager. Currently, she is a guest professor at the Faculty of Medical Sciences of Santa Casa de São Paulo, where she discusses socio-critical approaches to Public Mental Health Policies.

Elise Bromann Bukhave is a senior lecturer based in the Occupational Therapy Department at University College Absalon, Naestved. Elise holds a part-time position as postdoc at Roskilde University, Denmark. She has engaged in scholarship, teaching and writing on national and international levels for several years.

Ana Carreira De Mello is a Brazilian occupational therapist and PhD student at the Federal University of São Carlos, Brazil. She has training in the DOTM and Educational Processes in Health. Currently, she works in private practice with older adults in São Paulo, Brazil. Professional interests include occupational therapy and mental health, clinical reasoning, professional practice, oral history, epistemology and gerontology.

Jane Clewes qualified as an occupational therapist in 1983 and has since worked in the NHS in the UK, in mental health settings, including in generic/extended roles.

Sonia Maria Leonardi Ferrari is one of the founders and current board member of the Instituto A Casa de São Paulo, in Brazil, where she has been developing her clinical practice in mental health for over 40 years, advising beginning professionals and teaching about contemporary psychoses and pathologies. Sonia is one of the founders of the Centre for Specialties in Occupational Therapy (CETO) in which, in partnership with Jô Benetton, she coordinates the Clinical Training course in the DOTM.

Jill Maglio is an occupational therapist and founder of Holistic Circus Therapy and CircusAid. Jill has over 15 years of experience in using circus as an educational and community-building tool. Her involvement with circus research has been published in the *Australian Journal of Occupational Therapy*. She has been noted for her innovative work in combining social circus with occupational therapy to promote the acquisition of life skills among diverse populations.

Tais Quevedo Marcolino is an associate professor in the Occupational Therapy Department and Occupational Therapy Post-graduate Programme at the Federal University of São Carlos, Brazil. Tais has clinical training in the DOTM. Her research areas are the DOTM, adult mental health, clinical/professional reasoning, reflective practice and collaborative methodologies, including professional development through communities of practice.

Anri-Louise Oosthuizen is a South African occupational therapist. She is the founder and CEO of the NGO Growing the Nations Therapy Programmes. She played a pivotal role in the establishment of occupational therapy in Madagascar, including under- and post-graduate curriculum development, lecturing, service establishment and capacity building. She specialises in paediatrics, sensory integration and community development.

Kate Sherry is a South African occupational therapist with a focus on rural and remote community practice and service development. She has worked in South Africa, Madagascar and Tristan da Cunha (among other places), combining hands-on occupational therapy with research, teaching, advocacy and health systems strengthening.

Foreword

On a sunny day in Eastbourne, September 2017, *Diverse Roles for Occupational Therapists*, our multiauthor volume published by M&K Publishing, was launched at the second national conference for occupational therapists working in diverse settings, hosted at the University of Brighton. Working in diverse settings is an area of increasing interest for occupational therapists as their added value is being sought in an expanding range of settings. Accordingly, the idea for our book arose out of a desire to collect knowledge and experience from a band of practitioners in diverse and extended roles and to present them in a way that would be easily accessible and practical, to help occupational therapists explore and better understand practice in a range of professional roles beyond their own fields. The book captured honest accounts, combining descriptions of occupational therapists' day-to-day processes with case studies set against a backdrop of differing service structures and demands.

The conference had secured Jennifer Creek as one of its speakers and we took the opportunity to listen to Jennifer's engaging address. Jennifer, in turn, heard our sales pitch as we introduced our book, its developmental journey and its purpose. Following our presentation, Jennifer approached us and expressed genuine interest in the book. To our surprise, she inquired whether we would be interested in collaborating with her on developing a follow-up volume. We were and, as we discussed the possibilities, it felt important for us that a second volume would need to return to what we saw as the profession's sociologically based roots, to connect social theory with practice. By exploring occupational therapy in diverse settings from a more theoretical perspective, situating the discourse within a wider historical and societal context, we hoped to invite readers to consider their own practice theories and how these have the potential to inform and shape their role, as the profession moves into the future.

Enter stage left, Nick Pollard. Nick had been a great guide and support to us (Jane and Rob) in navigating some of the perils and pitfalls of editing a large volume. We had initially approached Nick for advice about securing the right publisher for the project; and Nick subsequently wrote a generous foreword for us, in which he described his own experiences and the questions that these had raised as he navigated his own professional practice. We were thrilled when Nick responded with such enthusiasm to being part of this follow-up project. Nick brought with him a vision for a book that would bring together occupational therapy and occupational science theory, with social theories being situated more recognisably within our professional field. By critically examining these shared narratives, Nick suggested, we might develop a discourse that would speak to and inform occupational therapy students and practitioners alike. We hoped to promote a deeper exploration of theory in our own work-based communities, as well as establishing stronger connections between our theories and those of other professions.

Over the next two years, with all the enthusiasm that comes with the early blue sky stages of a new project, we met for a series of summits at the British Library, discussing our ideas and concerns. We hammered out the shape of a book that we hoped would broaden the theoretical landscape of our profession and galvanise new connections with ongoing developments in social practice, as it was being articulated through the social practice theory discourse.

The treatment of occupational therapy as social practice seeks to collapse the hierarchical nature of knowledge, meaning and social institutions per se and, instead, allow all aspects of the practices that constitute occupational therapy to be considered and compared to similar practices across other fields and disciplines. Such deconstruction provides the flexibility to explore activity and occupation, their purposes and their functions, in new ways.

Through this new, thoughtful and provoking volume, the authors use the social practice perspective to gain fresh insight into our profession's historical, current and future developments. They explore ways in which occupational therapists have shaped and adapted their own practice to meet the needs of other social practice spheres; both those of the institutions in which the practice of occupational therapists occurs and those of the individuals and communities engaging with occupational therapy as recipients. The authors bring a theoretical perspective to bear when looking at the means by which occupational therapists address diverse concerns across ever-increasing practice settings, tailoring their contributions to the demands of local contexts and institutional structures of practice. These practices encapsulate the choices people make about how and where to participate in activities and connect them across a diverse network of structures and settings. The more we learn to see our own practice through this lens, the greater our capacity to challenge limiting barriers and promote opportunities to cross boundaries.

Jennifer and Nick worked onwards with the book and drew in the contributors and authors of various chapters. This has produced a book that captures different voices, experiences and interpretations. It is anticipated that the conversations the book generates, and will continue to generate as it reaches a wider audience, have game-changing potential for a profession that is continuing to grow and develop its understanding of the connectedness of all that holds meaning for us and our communities in our ever-changing world, through shared social practices.

Jane Clewes and Robert Kirkwood

Preface

In the 21st century, change in health and social care systems is a continuous feature of the practice environment of occupational therapists and other professional groups. Governments all over the world need to demonstrate their capacity to manage spending on health and social care services against their ability to meet population needs. World health policies demonstrate growing concern over anticipated demographic change towards older populations with complex needs, combined with economic uncertainty, rising inequalities and climate change. In 2020, the COVID-19 pandemic demonstrated how easily services can be challenged, and even overwhelmed, by health events, even when they have been predicted and expected.

In order to survive and progress in this context, occupational therapists have to find ways of navigating the organisations within which and through which they work. Organisational systems and structures can sometimes appear fragmented and impenetrable so lines of accountability and responsibility are difficult to identify. Professional knowledge tends to be developed in silos and disseminated through privileged channels that are not accessible to all. The aim of this book is to help occupational therapy practitioners to make sense of these realities so that they not only feel good about the work they do but also know they are doing an effective job.

The overarching theme of the book is the ways in which occupational therapists around the world are creating spaces for healthy patterns of occupation to develop in diverse settings. Populations in these settings might include people living with structural poverty, refugees, people displaced by natural disasters, homeless people and those experiencing the intersection of more than one of these conditions. The book is intended to support the professional reasoning of occupational therapists working in such settings, outside mainstream health and social care services, to help them develop effective strategies and to promote professional resilience.

The book is designed to be practical and useful; for example, by making explicit the ways in which social rules shape and constrain practice so that the practitioner is better able to understand the impact that competing values and professional cultures have on what can be achieved. Throughout the text, real-life examples are given to show that professional reasoning includes finding pragmatic ways of dealing with real constraints on time and resources, as practitioners work towards the achievement of our professional goals. Strategies are offered for working in the grey areas of practice, acknowledging that occupational therapy does not operate in a black-and-white universe.

Social practice theory is offered as a useful and appropriate theory for understanding occupational therapy in diverse settings. Different aspects of occupational therapy are explored from this theoretical perspective, including the impact of managerialism on the profession, the space-times of practice, issues of access, resources and responding to change. Chapters are illustrated with examples of how this theory can inform and support practice outside mainstream health and social care services.

Contributors to the book have been drawn from countries in Europe, North America, South America and Africa, bringing a wealth of varied experience and expertise to the task of theorising occupational therapy practice in diverse settings. The book may be read from beginning to end but each chapter can also be read separately. Topics are cross-referenced in the text and there is a comprehensive index. A glossary of technical terms is provided at the end of the book.

Jennifer Creek and Nick Pollard

Acknowledgements

Nick Pollard would like to thank Linda, Joshua, Daisy and Olivia for their support and patience at home during the preparation of this book. He would also like to thank students and colleagues at Sheffield Hallam University College of Health, Wellbeing and Life sciences for their support.

1 History and early development of occupational therapy

Jennifer Creek and Michael Allen

Introduction

In developed countries, where occupational therapy has been established for many years, it is common to hear practice in mainstream health and social care settings described as 'traditional'. The implication is that the profession of occupational therapy grew out of health and social care services and has always had its home there. However, as this chapter demonstrates, the origins of the profession were much broader, encompassing a range of social movements and ideals.

The chapter is divided into four sections. The first section identifies some of the major social changes and social movements, mainly in Europe and North America, that contributed to the founding of the profession of occupational therapy at the beginning of the 20th century. The second section describes how occupational therapy developed in its early years, expanding professional practice, education and theory. Some of the major influences on that development are highlighted, including the impact of two World Wars and occupational therapy's close association with the medical profession. The third section offers an alternative understanding of how occupational therapy emerged as a profession, using a practice theory perspective. The final section outlines the theoretical perspective used in this chapter and throughout the book: social practice theory.

Origins of occupational therapy

It has been speculated that the roots of occupational therapy can be found in approaches to healthcare going back thousands of years (Levin 1938; Wilcock 2001). However, the profession of occupational therapy emerged in Great Britain and North America in the late 19th and early 20th centuries. This was a time of social reform, when attempts were being made in many industrialised countries to improve the lives of disadvantaged people, such as the urban poor, immigrants, women and those with mental illness. Several of the social and philosophical discourses prevalent at the time had an influence on the emergence and early development of the new profession of occupational therapy. Five of these discourses are discussed in this section: the women's movement, housing reform, the settlement movement, the arts and crafts movement and pragmatism.

Women's movement

Around the end of the 19th and beginning of the 20th centuries, in Europe and North America, a new class of young women, with an education and the right to own property,

DOI: 10.4324/9781003016755-1

found themselves with the potential to earn their own living or make an economic contribution to the household income (see Box 1.1 for how this change came about in the United Kingdom). To achieve this they needed 'professional training and employment opportunities' (Paterson 2010: 142). Most of the established male professions, such as medicine and the law, were closed to women, leading to the emergence of new, women's professions, such as housing management, nursing and therapeutic massage.

Box 1.1   Women's rights in the UK – 1800–1928

Throughout the 19th century, in Great Britain, the position of women in society was changing in response to more general socio-economic and political developments.

In 1800, women in Britain did not have the right to vote. Girls received less education than boys, were barred from universities and had access only to low-paid jobs: none of the established professions was open to women. A married woman had no way of supporting herself or her children, since anything she inherited or earned became the property of her husband. A man had the right to have sex with his wife, whether or not she agreed, and to force her to bear children, who then belonged to the father. Women tended to have many children because there was no certainty that they would all survive childhood. Births, marriages and deaths were registered by individual parishes and there was no central record of how many people were born and died.

During the 19th and early 20th centuries, a series of new laws was passed and enacted, giving more rights to women. The *Married Women's Property Act* of 1870 paved the way for the universal franchise by decreeing that wages and property earned by a married woman would be regarded as her own property, although any property she had brought into the marriage still belonged to her husband. In 1882, this principle was extended to include all women's property, regardless of its source. This meant that a woman could, in theory, live separately from her husband and have the means to support her children. The *Representation of the People Act* of 1918 gave the vote to women over the age of 30 who met minimum property qualifications. The *Representation of the People Act* of 1928 extended the voting franchise to all women over the age of 21, which meant that for the first time women had the vote on the same terms as men.

By the end of 1870, women had the right to education up to the tertiary level. The medical profession agreed to allow women to become doctors and the London School of Medicine for Women was set up in 1874. A women's college was established in Cambridge in 1880 and women were allowed to attend lectures, with permission and chaperonage, although they were not permitted to take degrees until 1920. By 1910, women could become accountants and bankers but not diplomats or lawyers.

In the United States, women could not be awarded a degree before 1831. The first woman to earn a medical degree, Elizabeth Blackwell, qualified in 1849 but was not allowed to practise because it was 'assumed women were morally unfit to practice medicine ... ignorant, inexact, untrustworthy, un-businesslike, lacking in sense and mental perception, and contemptuous of logic' (Khalsa, n.d.).

In Canada, women were able to earn university degrees from 1872 onwards but only a relatively small number of female university graduates went into traditionally male professions, such as medicine or law. While women with less education were more likely to go into domestic service, married middle-class women 'were expected to become members of philanthropic organizations such as the IODE [Imperial Order of the Daughters of the Empire]' (Friedland 2011: 10).

Some women acted as trailblazers, introducing to others the potential for pursuing a professional career, often as an alternative to marriage. In the United Kingdom, one of these women was Octavia Hill, born in 1838, who is probably best remembered as one of the founders of the National Trust. Hill renovated and managed several housing estates in London for various bodies, including the Church of England. She employed young, unmarried women to act as housing managers, collecting rents on the estates and checking that tenants were looking after their homes. From these beginnings, housing management became an acceptable career for women (Darley 2010).

Housing reform

Through the mid to late 19th century, the industrialisation of the United Kingdom and the United States led to rapid population growth, especially in towns and cities. This placed stress on the infrastructure of cities, leading to urban poverty, shortage of decent housing, the growth of slums, high crime rates and the spread of diseases, such as typhoid and cholera (see Box 1.2). In addition to the physical dangers associated with poor housing, slum dwellers were considered to be at risk of moral degradation from the corrupting influence of overcrowding, filth, bad air, alcohol and profanity (von Hoffman 1998).

Box 1.2   Housing reform in the United Kingdom and the United States – 1848–1875

In the 19th century, overcrowding in expanding industrial cities, together with poor sanitation and lack of clean water, led to outbreaks of infectious diseases, such as cholera and typhoid. Following the publication of a number of reports on the living conditions in slums, and lobbying from various groups and individuals, governments were pressured to pass legislation to improve public health. For example, the first *Public Health Act* was passed in the United Kingdom in 1848, setting up a General Board of Health. This was followed by numerous other Acts to promote the health of urban populations, such as the 1875 *Public Health Act*, which required local authorities to provide water, drainage and sewage disposal in the towns.

In the second half of the 19th century, governments also legislated to improve housing for the working poor. In the United States, the first *Tenement House Act* was passed in 1867, setting minimum standards for sanitation and ventilation in multi-occupancy housing. In the United Kingdom, the *Artisans' and Labourers' Dwellings Improvement Act* of 1875 gave local authorities the power to buy slum areas for redevelopment. Local authorities took responsibility for clearing the slums while new houses were built by philanthropic organisations and housing associations, such as the Peabody Trust in London.

Pressure on governments to legislate for improvement of the urban environment came from influential individuals, such as Edwin Chadwick in Britain and Dr John H. Griscom in the United States (von Hoffman 1998). In London, Octavia Hill was prominent in pursuing housing reform, although she was against the idea of giving charity. Hill took on responsibility for the management of a number of properties, including the Red Cross Cottages, built by the Church of England to house the working poor in Southwark. One of the young women she employed was Elizabeth Casson, who became Secretary of the Red Cross Hall from 1908 to 1913 (https://victorianweb.org/art/architecture/homes/80.html) and who set up the first occupational therapy programme in the United Kingdom (Darley 2010).

Hill's philosophy was to provide good housing for poor people but only on the condition that they paid their rent and kept the property clean. She was as much concerned about the social and mental welfare of her tenants as their physical well-being. For example, when the Red Cross Cottages were built, Hill insisted that the estate should include gardens for recreation and a communal hall where tenants could receive education and enjoy various entertainments (Darley 2010).

Settlement house movement

Another young woman who worked in London with Octavia Hill was Henrietta Rowland, a social activist and reformer. Hill introduced Rowland to Samuel Barnett, a clergyman who also supported her work; the couple married in 1873 and went to live in Whitechapel, a deprived area of London (Wilcock 2001). The Barnetts shared a vision of how they could engage educated, middle-class young people in changing the lives of the poor by creating 'a place for future leaders to live and work as volunteers in London's East End, bringing them face to face with poverty, and giving them the opportunity to develop practical solutions that they could take with them into national life' (www.toynbeehall.org). In 1884, in fulfilment of this vision, the couple established the first settlement house, Toynbee Hall, in the East End of London, with 16 settlers (see Box 1.3). The Women's University Settlement, also located in London, supplied women for a wide range of social work positions, including housing managers for Octavia Hill.

Box 1.3 Settlement house movement – 1884

A settlement is simply a means by which men or women may share themselves with their neighbours; a club-house in an industrial district, where the condition of membership is the performance of a citizen's duty; a house among the poor, where residents may make friends with the poor.

(Barnett 1898: 26)

In 1884, Samuel and Henrietta Barnett founded the first of the settlement houses, Toynbee Hall (n.d.), in the east end of London, to offer amenities, education and guidance to people living in impoverished urban areas (Darley 2010). The basic rationale for Toynbee Hall was to narrow the gap between social classes by encouraging those with money and education to spend time among the poor.

In London, the Women's University Settlement was founded in 1887 by a number of individuals from the women's colleges at Cambridge and Oxford Universities. The objective was to 'promote the welfare of the poorer districts of London, more especially of the women and children, by devising and advancing schemes which tend to elevate them, and by giving them additional opportunities in education and recreation' (www.blackfriars-settlement.org.uk/history). Women from London colleges were invited to live at the Settlement rent free, in exchange for their work in the community.

The settlement house movement quickly spread to North America. Following a visit to Toynbee Hall, two American women, Jane Addams and Ellen Gates Starr, returned to the United States in 1889 and established Hull House Settlement in Chicago (Wilcock 2001: 388). Their intention was 'to integrate new immigrants into American society ... to provide a centre for the higher civic and social life, to institute and maintain educational and philanthropic enterprises and to investigate and improve the conditions in the industrial districts of Chicago' (Davis and McCree 1931, quoted in Paterson 2010: 7). The settlement movement continued to expand across the United States, ' ... with an international reputation for social welfare programmes [and] women's suffrage' (Paterson 2010: 7–8).

In Canada, settlement houses 'were established by concerned groups to address social problems resulting from poverty, industrial expansion, poor living conditions and the growing number of immigrants' (Friedland 2011: 8). The first one, Evangelia House, opened in Toronto in 1902 and by 1917 there were 13 in different parts of Canada, working mainly with immigrant populations 'to develop skills and knowledge, to build communities, and to improve the quality of life' (Friedland 2011: 53).

Arts and crafts movement

The arts and crafts movement began in Britain at the end of the 19th century, as a reaction against the dehumanising effects of industrialisation (see Box 1.4). The goal of the movement was to restore dignity to workers by giving them control over the process and quality of their work (Paterson 2010), but its influence extended beyond paid work to other aspects of the lives of poor people, such as education and aesthetics. The movement rapidly spread to other countries, including the United States and Canada.

Box 1.4   Arts and crafts movement – 1880–1920

The arts and crafts movement began in Britain and flourished in Europe and North America between about 1880 and 1920. The movement's leaders in Britain were two prominent thinkers of the late 19th century, John Ruskin and William Morris. Both men felt that factory work took away the knowledge and dignity once found in work, and alienated the worker from the product of his labours. They believed that, in contrast, people who engaged in handicrafts did not just make objects but also created themselves in the process (Sennett 2008).

John Ruskin was the leading British art critic of the Victorian era and was also influential in the sphere of social criticism. In 1860, he published a series of four essays in which he argued against the deleterious effects of capitalism and industrialism. 'That country is the richest which nourishes the greatest number of noble and happy human beings; that man is richest who, having perfected the function of his own life to the utmost, has always the widest helpful influence, both personal, and by means of his possessions, over the lives of others' (Ruskin 1862: 105). Ruskin helped to inspire the settlement movement; and the first settlement house, Toynbee Hall, was named after one of the young men who worked with him on social projects in Oxford (Hilton 2002).

William Morris was a successful textile designer, poet and novelist, who described himself as 'a practical Socialist' (Morris 1894: 93); someone who worked towards changing the social norms that created huge inequalities of wealth and opportunity. Morris and a group of his fellow students at Oxford were strongly influenced by the writings of Ruskin and developed his ideas into the arts and crafts movement.

One of the leaders of the arts and crafts movement in Britain, John Ruskin, was distressed by the overt inequalities within society and the appalling poverty of many working people. He used his writing and speaking to push for social reform in a number of areas: poverty, old age, women's rights, housing, education and employment (Friedland 2011). Ruskin supported Octavia Hill in her efforts to improve housing for the working poor, including lending her money to lease her first three houses (Darley 2010).

Another prominent member of the arts and crafts movement, William Morris, was concerned that factory work, in which each worker carried out only a part of the process of production, alienated the worker from what he was doing. Like Ruskin, Morris decried a society in which there were very rich and very poor people and wanted to use art 'as a means of educating and elevating the human spirit' (Friedland 2011: 36). Morris worked for a time in the late 1890s with George Barton, who became one of the founder members of the first national occupational therapy association in the United States, the National Society for the Promotion of Occupational Therapy (NSPOT) (Paterson 2010).

The Chicago Arts and Crafts Society, which was the first to be set up in the United States, was organised in 1897 at the settlement house, Hull House (Breines 1986), which was also associated with the American philosophy of pragmatism.

Pragmatism

In the late 19th century, several social and philosophical movements coalesced around Hull House and the University of Chicago. One of these philosophies was pragmatism (see Box 1.5), which has been described as 'the philosophy of "common sense", problem solving, activity, and adaptation, dimensions by which occupational therapists have traditionally bound themselves' (Breines 1986: 56).

Box 1.5   Pragmatism

The philosophy of pragmatism was first formulated by Charles Sanders Pierce in Cambridge, Massachusetts, in the early 1870s (Audi 1999) but is most closely associated with the University of Chicago and Hull House. Prominent exponents of pragmatism included John Dewey, George Herbert Mead and Jane Addams in Chicago, and William James at Harvard University.

Pragmatism has been described as 'the great American philosophy', which developed in response to 'the social currents of immigration to a new world, along with the influences of the Civil War [that] presented new problems which required creative solutions' (Breines 1986: 55).

Pragmatism focuses on the dynamic relationship between the individual, society and the environment. Human development is believed to proceed through the experiences people have throughout their lives with objects and individuals in the environment. Knowledge and truth are constantly revised as people learn from individual and collaborative experiences (Breines 1986). With their focus on the intersection of theory and practice, many pragmatists saw philosophising as an active process, 'often participating in experiments in education and working for egalitarian social reforms' (Whipps and Lake 2016).

Julia Clifford Lathrop, an eminent social reformer and advocate for women's rights, lived at Hull House for 22 years, from 1890, working closely with the two founders, Jane Addams and Ellen Gates Starr. Lathrop became the first woman member of the Illinois State Board of Control, in which capacity she visited many facilities, in and around Chicago, that 'collectively housed people who were mentally ill, aged, sick or disabled' (Social Welfare History Project 2011). From 1894, Lathrop worked with Graham Taylor, of the Chicago Commons Settlement House, to organise a series of social work lectures, which evolved into a year-long social work educational programme, based at the Chicago School of Civics and Philanthropy (University of Chicago School of Social Service Administration, n.d.).

While working for the State Board of Control, Lathrop toured the asylums in Illinois and saw for herself the stultifying boredom induced in patients by having to sit 'in idleness for hours together, their attendants satisfied with supplying their bodily needs and making no effort to rouse or stimulate them' (Friedland 2011: 26). She decided to see if training the asylum attendants would remedy the situation and, together with Rabbi Emil Gustave Hirsch, a social reformer who taught philosophy at the University of Chicago (Breines 1986), set up a six-week training course in *Occupations for Attendants in Mental Institutions* at the Chicago School of Civics and Philanthropy (Hopkins 1978).

One of the social work students who attended this course in 1911, Eleanor Clarke Slagle, went on to work at the Phipps Psychiatric Clinic at Johns Hopkins University, with psychiatrist Adolph Meyer. Lathrop, Hirsch, Meyer and Slagle were all involved in the mental hygiene movement, which started in the United States in 1908 with the aim of improving care and treatment in mental hospitals. The pragmatist philosopher, William James, was also involved with the movement. Slagle and Meyer became key figures in the early development of the occupational therapy profession.

Early development of occupational therapy

The previous section described some of the social movements that formed a context for the emergence of occupational therapy. This section looks at four processes by which occupational therapy has attempted to gain professional recognition and status: these are professionalisation, practice, education and theorising (Hugman 1991; Reed and Sanderson 1992).

Professionalisation

During the first half of the 20th century, occupational therapy progressed from its beginnings in the actions of social reformers in the United Kingdom and North America to become a recognised and regulated profession in many countries. Professionalisation has been described as a process through which an occupational group moves incrementally from partial professionalisation towards full professional status (Hugman 1991). This process takes place in stages, including the establishment of a professional association, agreement on professional standards, the development of professional training and consolidation of a specialist knowledge base, which together makes up the organising structure of the profession.

The beginning of the 20th century saw an increase in the number of occupational groups seeking some form of professional status, possibly as a response to a growing social and economic need for technical expertise (Schön 1983). Between 1894 and 1935, seven of the health and social care professions in the United Kingdom, which had all started as careers for educated, middle-class women, established their own professional bodies; among them occupational therapy (Paterson 2010).

The first professional body for occupational therapists was the National Society for the Promotion of Occupational Therapy (NSPOT), founded in 1917 in the United States (Wilcock 2002). Three of the founding members, Adolph Meyer, Eleanor Clarke Slagle and George Barton, were introduced in the previous section. In Canada, two regional professional associations were formed in 1920: the Canadian Society of Occupational Therapists of Manitoba and the Ontario Society of Occupational

Therapy. The first occupational therapy association in the United Kingdom was the Scottish Association of Occupational Therapy, established in 1932. The English professional body, the Association of Occupational Therapists, was formed in 1935. An international professional body, the World Federation of Occupational Therapists (WFOT), was inaugurated at a meeting in England in 1952 (Paterson 2010). The founder members were Australia, Canada, Denmark, India, Israel, New Zealand, South Africa, Sweden, the United Kingdom and the United States of America. Seven of these ten founding countries were Anglophone and five of them had been part of the British Empire in the 19th century. (The development of occupational therapy in Brazil, which started in 1946, is discussed in Chapters 8 and 9.)

Practice

In the early years of the 20th century, the first trained occupational therapists, practising in the United States, Canada and the United Kingdom, worked in three main areas: tuberculosis, physical rehabilitation and psychiatry.

Tuberculosis was a major cause of disability and death in the late 19th and early 20th centuries. Tuberculosis sanatoriums were established across Europe and North America to provide fresh air treatment that combined rest with graded exercise (Paterson 2010; Friedland 2011). This form of treatment, which was developed by medical practitioners, had a direct influence on occupational therapy in the United Kingdom and North America. In England, Dr Jane Walker, who founded the East Anglian Sanatorium, became a founding vice-president of the Association of Occupational Therapists (Wilcock 2002). In North America, Thomas Kidner, one of the founding members of the NSPOT and its president for six years, worked for the National Tuberculosis Association in New York.

Prior to the establishment of occupational therapy as a profession, handicrafts were employed in the rehabilitation of orthopaedic patients in hospitals and rehabilitation workshops. The teachers were called variously ward occupations aides (Canada), re-construction aides (USA) or instructors (Scotland). Thanks to the work of these people, by the time of the First World War, the use of activity as a therapeutic medium was familiar to many medical practitioners.

The emerging profession of occupational therapy gained medical recognition and increased public support from the work of rehabilitating war-wounded soldiers (Hopkins 1978; Paterson 2010). During the War, the numbers of wounded soldiers and the severity of their injuries created a huge demand for effective services to prepare as many as possible to return to the front line (Friedland 2011). As it became apparent that many soldiers would not recover fully from their injuries, services were designed to enable them to retrain and re-enter the workforce.

Many of the first generation of occupational therapists worked in psychiatric hospitals. In the United States, for example, Eleanor Clarke Slagle worked as director of the occupational therapy department at the Phipps Psychiatric Clinic in Baltimore, where Adolph Meyer was psychiatrist-in-chief (Hopkins 1978). Margaret Barr Fulton, who trained in the United States, became the first qualified occupational therapist to work in the United Kingdom, being employed at the Aberdeen Royal Asylum from 1925 until her retirement in 1963 (Paterson 2010). The growth of occupational therapy practice in psychiatric hospitals was promoted by some powerful psychiatrists, including Adolph Meyer in the United States, Sir David Henderson in Scotland and Alfred Thomas Hobbs in Canada.

It has been claimed that Meyer was 'not only the dominant figure in American psychiatry between 1895 and 1940, but one of the two great figures who changed psychiatry into ... a discipline that affords meaningful insights into human behavior' (Lidz 1966/1985: 35), The author did not say who the other great figure was. Meyer, together with Eleanor Clarke Slagle, developed a method of treating psychiatric patients based on the work of the pragmatist philosopher, William James (1899/2008), which Slagle called 'habit training' (Reed and Sanderson 1980: 190).

Education

The first group of women to complete a specialist training course and be given the title of *Occupational Therapist* attended the Favill School of Occupational Therapy at the Chicago School of Civics and Philanthropy, in the United States, which was founded in 1915 (Friedland 2003). More occupational therapy schools were set up in the United States in 1918, when the US Army Surgeon General requested that new centres 'be established to train reconstruction aides in the treatment and rehabilitation of physically and mentally traumatised soldiers' (Paterson 2010: 86–87). The first occupational therapy training programme in Canada was established in 1926, at the University of Toronto, where the curriculum was adapted from 'the best curricula in the United States' (Friedland 2003: 167).

In 1926, Dr Elizabeth Casson (who, as a young woman, had worked with Octavia Hill, see above) visited the occupational therapy department at Bloomingdale Hospital, in New York, and the Boston School of Occupational Therapy. This trip gave her the idea of starting an occupational therapy school in England (Casson 1950). Casson opened the Dorset House School of Occupational Therapy in 1930, at her private psychiatric clinic in Bristol.

The first Principal of Dorset House, Constance Tebbit, trained at the Philadelphia School of Occupational Therapy, where Fulton had received her qualification. The Philadelphia School was one of several set up in 1918, and both Slagle and Kidner lectured on the occupational therapy programme there. The first occupational therapy training programme in Scotland began in 1937, at the Astley Ainslie Institution in Edinburgh. The curriculum was based 'as closely as possible upon the Occupational Therapy course at the University of Toronto' (Macdonald 1939: 19).

The syllabus agreed on by training courses in the United States, Canada and the United Kingdom was in roughly three parts (AOT 1968), as shown in Table 1.1.

As national professional associations were formed, one of their functions was to establish minimum standards for occupational therapy education within each country. In 1958, the WFOT produced an international programme for the education of occupational therapists (Mendez 1986), which, in 1971, became the *Recommended Minimum Standards for the Education of Occupational Therapists* (WFOT 2016). Any professional occupational therapy association wishing to become a full member of the WFOT must establish at least one programme of education in their country that meets these minimum standards.

Table 1.1 The occupational therapy curriculum (AOT 1968)

The body and mind in normal health; deficiency, disease and trauma	Much of this part of the curriculum was designed and delivered by medical doctors and psychologists.
Occupations and techniques and their use as a treatment	Students learned a number of crafts and other activities to a level of proficiency. The theoretical component of this part of the syllabus, which can be seen as the specialist knowledge base of the profession, included the principles of using activity in the treatment of various mental and physical disorders, the characteristics of different activities and the therapeutic process.
Clinical experience	Students were required to undertake a range of supervised practical experience in both physical and psychiatric healthcare settings.

Theorising

The range of influences on occupational therapy at its foundation was broad and eclectic. As outlined above, some of the origins of the profession can be found in various movements for social reform, such as women's rights, housing reform and 'common sense psychiatry' (Lidz 1966/1985: 43), and in the philosophy of pragmatism. However, the emerging profession soon aligned itself with medicine and retreated from the social activism of its founders: ' ... within a few short years, the engineers, teachers, architects, social workers, artists, and vocational educators who had been so involved with occupational therapy early on had withdrawn and prominent medical men had taken over' (Friedland 2011: 152).

By the end of the First World War, there was a general acceptance that any form of medical treatment should be 'established on scientific lines' (O'Sullivan 1955: xi). Since occupational therapy did not, at that time, have an agreed scientific or other theoretical basis, this was provided by the medical profession. The pragmatic approach of the first occupational therapists was largely replaced by 'the acquisition of techniques and the description of programs' (Serrett 1985: 20), as doctors not only took responsibility for guiding practice but also exerted intellectual control:

> Occupational therapy [adopted] the rationality of the medical model with its focus on pathology. Its systematic approach to wholesome, healthy living as seen in the processing of competency behaviours was replaced with the narrow perspective of the medical model ... Its epistemological base shifted from the social sciences to the functional requirements of the physical sciences and focus on the minute and measurable.
>
> (Shannon 1977: 231)

The knowledge base of the profession included both theoretical and applied knowledge, as shown in the curricula of the first occupational therapy educational programmes in the United States, Canada and the United Kingdom (Table 1.1). From the first, it was clear that the physician would 'supply the beliefs, philosophies, and principles of occupational therapy' (Serrett 1985: 20) while the occupational therapist would implement the programmes they designed.

This section and the preceding one outlined the emergence and development of occupational therapy as described in published occupational therapy histories (e.g., Wilcock 2001, 2002; Paterson 2010; Friedland 2011). The next section offers an alternative way of viewing the foundation and ongoing development of the profession, using social practice theory to structure an understanding of why and how occupational therapy came into being.

An alternative perspective

When the history of occupational therapy is described from a social practice perspective, it becomes possible to see that the profession came into existence through links formed between the ideas and aspirations of certain groups of people, the materials and resources available at the time and the skills, knowledge and technical competence of early practitioners. The necessary elements of occupational therapy were already in place and, once they were connected, the emergence of the new profession became inevitable.

This section is divided into two parts. The first explores the elements and conditions that brought about the emergence of occupational therapy in the early 20th century, including the beliefs and intentions of key, influential people, the knowledge and skills of practitioners and the resources available to them. The second part employs a social practice theory lens to explain how occupational therapy emerges from and is embedded in a web of social practices.

How occupational therapy came into existence

By the end of the 19th century, in wealthy, industrialised countries such as the United Kingdom and the United States, the daughters of middle-class parents could attain the same level of education as their brothers (Box 1.1), although they were expected to marry rather than earn their own living. The world of work was considered to be the province of men, while women were thought to belong in the domestic sphere. Women were barred from many of the established, male professions of the time, such as the law and diplomacy, and their access to other professions was not on equal terms with men. The desire of women to use their education and talents in a wider field than the home, in conjunction with strictly limited opportunities to enter the established male professions, led to the emergence of several new professions that brought women's domestic skills into the public sphere.

These new professions provided an outlet for young, educated women to utilise their active minds, in conjunction with their caring and nurturing skills, in meeting a variety of social needs. Many of these needs arose from the conditions brought about by industrialisation; such as inadequate housing, child labour, long working hours and economic migration. Women sought to alleviate the conditions afflicting the poor by working as, for example, teachers, nurses, housing managers and social workers. Occupational therapy is one of the women's professions that came into being in this way, in the early 21st century.

Some of the roots of occupational therapists' beliefs and values can be traced to the social movements described above, through individuals who were active in them and who had direct links with the founders of the profession. For example, the housing reform movement was connected with occupational therapy through Octavia Hill and Elizabeth

Casson; the settlement house movement through Henrietta Barnett, Jane Addams and Ellen Gates Starr; the arts and crafts movement through John Ruskin, Octavia Hill and George Barton, and pragmatism through Julia Clifford Lathrop, Adolph Meyer and Eleanor Clark Slagle, amongst others. All these people were social activists and reformers, who sought to improve the lives of disadvantaged people in society: the poor, immigrants, working-class women and people with mental illnesses. Their ideas and aspirations continued to be translated into action by the first occupational therapy practitioners.

In order to implement practical solutions to the social problems they identified, Hill, Addams and other reformers employed young, educated men and women to work as housing managers, social workers, aides and instructors in various settings. These young workers brought their knowledge, skills and motivation to bear in devising pragmatic solutions to the difficulties of everyday life experienced by disadvantaged groups. Women found that their domestic skills could be utilised in a wider social sphere; observing, advising, educating, instructing, mentoring and supporting. Thus, the connection was made between the aspirations of leading social reformers and the skills of young women, who would become the first occupational therapists.

The emerging profession of occupational therapy also had close links to medicine and was promoted by some of the leading physicians of the time, who understood the value of occupation in the treatment of various disorders. These physicians included: Adolph Meyer and David Henderson in the field of psychiatry; Thomas Kidner and Robert Jones in orthopaedic medicine, and Jane Walker and Robert W. Philip in the treatment of tuberculosis, among others. Ward aides and instructors were skilled in craftwork and in teaching practical activities but were not expected to understand the principles of medical treatment and rehabilitation (Haworth and MacDonald 1948). They worked under the supervision of medical practitioners, who prescribed programmes of activity that were then carried out by the instructors. Thus, in the field of healthcare, the connection between a medical practitioner and activity instructor placed propositional knowledge about the therapeutic potential of activity with the doctor and procedural knowledge of how to teach crafts with the proto-occupational therapist.

The settings in which occupational therapy came into existence were linked to the fields in which reformers, activists and practitioners operated. In turn, the resources available to proto-occupational therapists were part of these settings. Housing managers, such as Elizabeth Casson, visited tenants in their own homes. In addition to collecting rent, they went into the houses to check if any repairs were needed, observe whether or not children were attending school and find out if anyone in the family was sick (Darley 2010). All the estates managed by Octavia Hill had communal halls or rooms, where tenants could meet for education or entertainment, and there were outdoor spaces, such as gardens or children's playgrounds.

In the settlement houses, educated men and women lived and worked alongside the people they were trying to help. The houses were 'located within the impoverished communities they intended to serve' (Friedland 2011: 44) so that workers, whether voluntary or paid, saw at first-hand the conditions in which poor people lived and how they managed their daily lives.

In contrast, women who were employed as occupations aides, reconstruction aides or instructors worked in a variety of healthcare settings; including the infirmary wards of workhouses, tuberculosis sanatoriums, rehabilitation workshops, mental asylums, orthopaedic wards, military hospitals, convalescent centres for injured soldiers and 'institutions for the mentally defective' (Paterson 2010: 72). What all these settings had in common is that people lived in them for the duration of their treatment, while staff came into work for set hours. This meant that the occupations aides and instructors did not work with people in their usual living and working environments but saw them only as patients in the medical environment. The materials and resources available to these practitioners were those provided by the employing organisation rather than the everyday objects of people's lives.

At the time when occupational therapy was first emerging as a profession, Great Britain still had an Empire that extended around the globe. Power, privilege and authority were concentrated in the administrative structures of the Empire. Goods, wealth, raw materials and labour flowed from the colonies to Britain, leaving a global legacy of inequality that persists. In exchange, the colonies received laws, knowledge, education and technology, most of which were intended to benefit British rule and the continuance of exploitative and extractive trades, often despite the knowledge of the colonised populations. These actions were carried by traders, missionaries, administrators and their wives to the furthest reaches of the Empire, and justified by misrepresentation of colonised populations in culture, religion and science (Tharoor 2018; Sivasundaram 2021). Consequently, the colonisers believed that their ways of understanding and ordering the world were superior to those of the people they governed and that everyone benefited from the civilising influence of colonial rule (New World Encyclopaedia 2020). But their dominance went further, in that they 'exercised power and reinforced domination by establishing the parameters of permissible thinking and by suppressing challenging ideas' (Hammell 2011: 28).

With this colonial heritage and context, it was inevitable that the two countries where occupational therapy was first recognised, Great Britain and its most powerful former colony, the United States, would see themselves as the privileged and authoritative centre of the profession. Throughout the 20th century, occupational therapy was exported from these two countries, by their colonising governments, taking with them their own ways of understanding and practising;; in a process of 'theoretical imperialism [,] by which theorists develop and perpetuate theories that privilege their own perspectives while overlooking, ignoring or silencing the perspective of others' (Hammell 2011: 28). Like earlier colonialists, these occupational therapists believed implicitly that their knowledge and skills were superior to those of people in colonised countries. The flow of knowledge and experience was unidirectional, from the dominant to the subjugated nations, and English was established as the universal language of the profession before it was established in other countries.

How occupational therapy is structured

The practice of occupational therapy can be summed up as what occupational therapists do, but viewing occupational therapy through a practice theory lens reveals the structure that underpins and supports professional activities. Without a structure, there are just activities, dispersed over time and space, that can be performed by anyone. What occupational therapists do can be called occupational therapy because it is based on:

1   shared understandings of what is done
2   rules, principles, precepts and instructions for how it should be done
3   the reasons why it is done, that is, the ends and purposes of occupational therapy
     (Schatzki 1996).

These three structuring elements came together in the early 20th century, enabling the profession of occupational therapy to take shape. By the beginning of the century, firm connections had been made between the aspirations and skills of educated, middle-class women, the ideas of social and medical reformers and the places where those ideas were put into practice. As the century progressed, some of these links were strengthened, while others weakened and new connections continued to be made.

Before the onset of the First World War, occupations were being used in settlement houses and the community centres of housing estates 'as a means of creating social change through interaction, activities and education' (Friedland 2011: 48); and in hospitals, rehabilitation centres and asylums, 'to gain from the patient the desired physical function and/ or mental response' (Fulton, quoted in Paterson 2010: 40). The outbreak of hostilities, in 1914, saw an increased demand for the rehabilitation of injured soldiers and led to military hospitals and curative workshops being set up in Great Britain, Canada and France.

When the United States entered the War, in 1917, the Medical Department of the United States Army established 25 new training programmes for reconstruction aides, who would 'teach various forms of simple handcraft to patients in military hospitals and other sanitary formations of the Army, especially to those patients in the orthopaedic and surgical wards as well as patients suffering from nervous and mental diseases' (Medical Department 1918, p. 2, quoted in Low 1992: 38). Thus, a new link was made, between the practice of occupational therapy and the military.

Armies are large and powerful organisations, especially during wartime. In Britain, Europe and North America, military demands, standards and ways of working were given priority over other areas in which occupational therapists had been working. The principles and processes of rehabilitation, which had been developed by doctors and enacted by occupations aides, were systematised to improve efficiency, in order to return wounded soldiers as rapidly as possible to active service. 'The result was an orthopaedic system, organised in the same way as a scientifically managed factory' (Paterson 2010: 47).

To increase the efficiency of rehabilitation, experts in scientific management were brought in to advise army surgeons; and their methods of analysing and adapting activities, modifying environments and conserving energy were incorporated into the occupational therapy curriculum (Creighton 1992). The scientific management precept of changing the task to fit the man developed into the occupational therapy compensatory frame of reference (Paterson 2010).

The first two schools of occupational therapy in Britain were located within hospitals: a physical convalescent hospital in Scotland and a psychiatric clinic in England. The 25 courses set up in the United States during the First World War were located in colleges but were accredited by the American Medical Association, and students undertook their fieldwork practice in hospitals. In Canada, occupational therapy education was established in universities, with students having fieldwork placements and internships in hospitals, asylums, sanatoriums and curative workshops (Friedland 2011).

The first professional association of occupational therapists, the NSPOT, was set up just before America entered the First World War in 1917. All other occupational therapy associations were established after the War, when the profession had become more closely aligned with medicine. Doctors were closely involved in all these professional associations and, when the profession became regulated by the state, took a major role in the regulation process.

Thus, at the point in time when occupational therapy was named as a distinct entity, the medical profession was in a position to determine the professional role of occupational therapists, including what they could and could not do and the conditions of their being allowed to practise. In Schatzki's (1996) words, occupational therapists lost the power to:

1   create their own shared understandings of what they do
2   establish their own rules, principles and precepts for how it should be done
3   determine their own ends and purposes.

A Canadian occupational therapy historian, Judith Friedland wondered whether it had been a conscious, tactical decision, taken by occupational therapists to seek powerful allies in order to help to get the profession started, that led to the unintended consequence of 'giving over control of their destiny to physicians' (2011: 152).

It can be seen from this account that occupational therapy does not exist in isolation but is intimately connected with a range of other social practices that influence how society constructs occupational therapy. One of these constructions locates the profession, along with other health and social care professions, as a bulwark to protect the status quo against the threats and contamination of the poor and precarious in society.

This section has discussed how certain resources, competences and meanings, related to the needs of disadvantaged people in society, gradually coalesced into the practice of occupational therapy. In the process, occupational therapy became distinct from other practices, such as housing reform and social work, which initially shared some of those resources, competences and meanings. In part, occupational therapy evolved to separate from its social roots by aligning itself with the medical profession and relocating its activities from people's living spaces into hospital settings. In doing so, it gave up much of the power to determine its own purpose and functions.

The next section explains how social practice is understood in the context of this book and outlines the main features of practice theories.

What are theories of social practice?

Social theorists use the term **practice theory** in two ways: first, as a collective term that subsumes a range of theories that take social practices as their main focus; and, second, as a singular term to describe any one of the theories subsumed within the collective term and taking social practices as their central unit of analysis (Sedlačko 2017: 48). Practice theorists are united by:

> [the] belief that such phenomena as knowledge, meaning, human activity, science, power, language, social institutions, and historical transformation occur within and are aspects or components of the *field of practices*. The field of practices is the total nexus of interconnected human practices.
>
> (Schatzki 2001: 2)

The term *social practice* (often shortened simply to *practice*), does not equate to, for example, the practice of occupational therapy, which connotes the exercise of the profession of occupational therapy (Shorter Oxford English Dictionary 2002), nor does it equate to *praxis*, which is 'the whole of human action (in contrast to theory and mere thinking)' (Reckwitz 2002: 250). Rather, practice theorists equate practice with the German word *praktik*, meaning 'a routinised type of behaviour' (Reckwitz 2002: 250).

Practice theorists take practices as the site where social life transpires (Schatzki 2002), which leads to an ontological understanding of all social phenomena in terms of practices (Schatzki 2016). Such an ontology is necessarily flat, since a social world composed of practices has a single level, that of the field of practices (Schatzki 2016). The adoption of a flat ontology differentiates practice theory from theories that necessitate at least two levels of social reality by making a distinction between social structures and human agency (Schatzki 2016: 34). By shifting such phenomena as knowledge, meaning and social institutions into the sphere of practices, practice theory collapses the hierarchical notion that the social world is bifurcated into human agents and systemic structures. According to Giddens' theory of structuration (1984), systemic structures and human agency have a recursive relationship that continuously constructs and reproduces social life: 'The basic domain of study of the social sciences, according to the theory of structuration, is neither the experience of the individual actor, nor the existence of any form of societal totality, but social practices ordered across space and time' (Giddens 1984: 2).

This way of thinking about social life allows all social phenomena to be studied as aspects of social practices and the relationships between them. In recent years, the challenge of doing so has been taken up by theorists in what has become known as the practice turn in social theory (Schatzki 2001). The practice turn encompasses a plurality of fields, including philosophy, cultural studies, sociology and science and technology studies (Schatzki 2001).

The main features of practice theories

This section introduces and explains four of the key concepts found in theories of social practice: the concept of practice; the elements of practice; practice-as-performance/practice-as-entity, and teleoaffective structures. Other concepts are introduced in relevant chapters throughout the book.

Conceptualising a practice

As mentioned above, the central concept that links all practice theories is social practice. Practices are social constructs, defined and delimited by the scholar or researcher to meet specific ends, and have no objective reality. This means that they can be defined in a number of ways and conceived at multiple scales:

> There are different ways of delimiting "a" practice ... For example, some might consider smoking as part of other more encompassing practices such as "working", or "going out" or "taking a break". Others might treat each of the actions of which smoking is made (for example, rolling, lighting and inhaling) as separate practices, consequently viewing smoking as a complex or bundle of practices. Different routes make sense depending on the purpose of the enquiry and the analytic strategy that follows.
>
> (Blue et al. 2014: 39)

This flexibility makes practice theory a useful theory for studying occupational therapy at all levels, from the daily activities of the practitioner to the social purpose and function of the profession. Occupational therapists are familiar with the idea of human action at different scales. When looking at a simple task, such as rolling a cigarette, we can think of **practice-as-activity**. When looking at practices involving multiple activities, such as working, we can think of **practice-as-occupation**.

Some practice theorists are concerned with larger systems of practice, such as organisations (Nicolini 2012), everyday life (Shove et al. (2012) and human-technology relations (Morley 2017). Different terms are used to refer to how practices come together in wider groupings, such as assemblages, bundles, complexes, constellations, knots, networks and nexuses (Blue et al. 2014; Hui et al. 2017; Nicolini and Monteiro 2017), and there is no general agreement about when to use one rather than another. In this book, the term **constellation** is used to refer to a number of interdependent practices coming together as a system; so that the profession of occupational therapy is described as a constellation of practices that come together in contextually specific ways. For example, an occupational therapy clinician and an occupational therapy educator perform different practices but they are both parts of the constellation of occupational therapy.

Social practices never exist in isolation but always in relation to other practices; 'bound by happening in the same time and place or being bound together in harmonious or conflicting relationships' (Nicolini and Monteiro 2017: 4). This close interdependence means that the effects of a change in one practice 'ripple through the connections, affecting the [other] practice[s]' (Nicolini and Monteiro 2017: 5).

Despite there being multiple possibilities for defining the limits and scale of social practice, the authors and editors of this book have attempted to be consistent in how they conceptualise practice. Schatzki conceived of practices as composed of 'doings/sayings, tasks and projects' (Schatzki 2002: 74), which are separate from but intrinsically linked to material arrangements. Social life, he argued, 'inherently transpires as part of nexuses of practices and material arrangements' (Schatzki 2010: 129).

Schatzki's conception of a practice has points of commonality with Vygotsky's conception of activity, in that Vygotsky made a similar distinction between the immaterial and material elements of activities. He held that activity is the interface (similar to Schatzki's nexus) between the inner world of the individual and the outer physical and social worlds (Nicolini 2012). This means that, as with structure and agency in structuration theory, mental constructs and physical materials have a recursive relationship in which the mental affects the material and vice versa.

The elements of practice

For Reckwitz (2002: 249), practices have seven elements, 'forms of bodily activities, forms of mental activities, "things" and their use, a background knowledge in the form of understanding, know-how, states of emotion and motivational knowledge'. Shove and colleagues (2012) simplified this formulation to three elements: meanings, materials and competences. It is this less elaborate understanding of social practice, as being composed of meanings, materials and competences, that is adopted in this book.

According to Shove and colleagues, **meaning** is 'the social and symbolic significance of participation [in a practice] at any one moment' (Shove et al. 2012: 23). The social meaning of an activity derives from the purpose and value the activity has within a particular culture. The personal meaning of an activity is linked to the individual's goals and identity.

Materials include 'objects, infrastructures, tools, hardware and the body itself' (Shove et al. 2012: 23). They are the physical components of a person's life that are essential to the performance of all activities, not just making things.

Competence is defined as 'multiple forms of understanding and practical knowledgeability' (Shove et al. 2012: 23). People need to learn skills and knowledge in order to be able to perform activities successfully.

The three elements of practices 'are mutually shaping' (Shove et al. 2012: 32), in that each element exists in dynamic relation to the others: the particular constitution of each element is how it is because of the composition of the other two elements. Meanings, materials and competences coalesce in the moment of doing, giving rise to a social practice.

The process of combining and recombining elements to form different practices is complex since each element is comprised of multiple things. For example, patchwork quilting might involve: materials, such as needles, threads, scissors, fabric and sewing boxes; competences, such as the dexterity to cut fabric to the desired shape, to visualise the end product or to use a sewing machine, and meanings, such as ideas of relaxation, good ways to spend leisure time and what a good quilt is. This multiplicity of materials, meanings and competences combines in myriad ways during different moments of performance and in different contexts, making each performance a unique expression of the practice (see Hui 2012 for a practice theory analysis of how the materiality of patchwork quilting is affected by the mobility of practitioners).

Practice-as-performance/Practice-as-entity

Practices exist both in the moment of performance and between and beyond individual performances. Schatzki (1996) called these two modes of existence **practice-as-performance** and **practice-as-entity**. Practice-as-performance pertains to a practice in the moment of doing, that is to say, when a practice is being performed by a practitioner. For example, when someone is driving, the meanings, materials and competences of driving are combined by the practitioner in a particular time and space to create a discrete instance of driving.

A practice, however, is more than an individual performance or even the sum total of all performances past, present and future. Practices persist across space and time as well as in space and time. Schatzki identified that practices exist as entities or 'temporally unfolding and spatially dispersed nexus[es] of doings and sayings' (Schatzki 1996: 89). In other words, practice entities endure between moments of enactment because of the repeated reproduction of practice performances in multiple space-times. An example of this is the clapping games of children, that have endured across the world for hundreds of years, albeit in different and changing forms. While practice entities are derived from practice performances, the concept of practice-as-entity explains how practices can continue to exist even if they are not being performed in any given time and space: for example, driving continues to exist as a practice entity even if no one, anywhere in the world, performs the practice on a given day. Practice-as-entity also refers to how a practice continues to exist for individual practitioners between their own moments of performance: 'I am an occupational therapist even when I am not practising occupational therapy'.

Teleoaffective structures

Social practices are future-oriented in that they are performed with some outcome or outcomes in mind. The idea of practice histories, contributing to the organising and ordering of social practices through goal-oriented practice performances, is captured in the concept of **teleoaffective structures**. These structures are composed of 'ends, projects, tasks, purposes, beliefs, emotions and moods' (Schatzki 1996: 89), which help to organise and order practices in time and space. They guide and structure the range of possibilities for practice performances, based on the normative history of the practice. For example, the game of soccer has developed its own rules, norms, standards and expected outcomes that are different from those of other team sports. The emotional or affective quality of these structures comes from the idea that certain outcomes are more desirable or correct than others.

Teleoaffective structures indicate to practitioners how a practice should be performed: what needs to be or can be done; what order things need to be done in, and what outcomes are desirable (Nicolini 2012). When driving a bus, for example, the performer must use a range of accepted rules and techniques that distinguish driving a bus from similar practices, such as driving a private car. The finished product of a practice must be recognisable in terms of the desired outcome, with the success of the practice performance being judged by how well the finished product matches the desired outcome or the specifications and standards set for the practice.

Teleoaffective structures are not to be thought of as a deterministic, ordering force (Nicolini 2012); they are properties of practices and should not be conflated with the ends, goals or desires that are consciously formulated by individual practitioners. As Nicolini (2012: 167) pointed out, 'the teleo-affective structure [of a practice] only contributes by shaping what it makes sense to do'. In fact, 'determining which ends, projects, and emotions are obligatory or mandatory is open-ended' (Nicolini 2012: 167).

Conceptualising practices using Shove's three elements helps to capture this idea more clearly, since the various aspects of teleoaffectivity (ends, projects, tasks, purposes, beliefs, emotions and moods) are subsumed within the meaning element of practice. This simplifying move makes it clear that meaning is part of a practice and 'not something that stands outside or that figures as a motivational or driving force' (Shove et al. 2012: 24). As the various aspects of the meaning of a practice change, so the practice evolves in relation to the other practice elements, via moments of performance. However, change always occurs through the internal, dynamic relations of practice elements rather than the conscious decisions of autonomous practitioner-actors.

Summary and conclusion

The chapter explored the history and development of the occupational therapy profession in two ways. First, written records of the profession were mined to produce a chronological account of how the profession came into being and to identify key social influences on its development during the 20th century. Second, a practice theory lens was turned on that history to create an alternative understanding of how occupational therapy emerged, both out of and in relation to other social practices. The chapter finished with a brief description of the main features of practice theory, with some definitions of key concepts as they are used in this book. Further details of the theory are given in the relevant chapters throughout the book.

References

Association of Occupational Therapists (1968) Information on proferssional prospects and regulations governing membership of the association and an outline of the syllabus of course leading to the diploma. London: AOT.

Audi, R. (1999) *The Cambridge dictionary of philosophy*, 2nd edition. Cambridge: Cambridge University Press.

Barnett, S. (1898) University settlements. Online at https://infed.org/mobi/university-settlements/. Accessed May 2022.

Blackfriars Settlement (n.d.) Our history. Online at www.blackfriars-settlement.org.uk/history. Accessed May 2022.

Blue, S., Shove, E., Carmona, C., and Kelly, M.P. (2014) Theories of practice and public health: Understanding (un)healthy practices. *Critical Public Health*, 26(1): 36–50.

Breines, E. (1986) *Origins and adaptations: a philosophy of practice*. Lebanon, NJ: Geri-Rehab. Inc.

Casson, E. (1950) Foreword. In: B. Collins (ed.) *The story of the Dorset House School of Occupational Therapy 1930-1946*. Private publication. 1–4.

Creighton, C. (1992) The origin and evolution of activity analysis. *American Journal of Occupational Therapy*, 46(1): 45–48.

Darley, G. (2010) *Octavia Hill: social reformer and founder of the National Trust*. London: Francis Boutle.

Friedland, J. (2003) Muriel drive memorial lecture: why crafts? influences on the development of occupational therapy in Canada from 1890 to 1930. *Canadian Journal of Occupational Therapy*, 70(4): 204–212.

Friedland, J. (2011) *Restoring the spirit: the beginnings of occupational therapy in Canada, 1890–1930*. Montreal: McGill-Queen's University Press.

Giddens, A. (1984) *The constitution of society: outline of the theory of structuration*. Cambridge: Polity Press.

Hammell, K.W. (2011) Resisting theoretical imperialism in the disciplines of occupational science and occupational therapy. *British Journal of Occupational Therapy*, 74(1): 27–33.

Haworth, N.A., and MacDonald, E.M. (1948) *Theory of occupational therapy*. London: Ballière, Tindall and Cox.

Hilton, T. (2002) *John Ruskin*. New Haven: Yale University Press.

Hopkins, H.L. (1978) An historical perspective on occupational therapy. In: H.L. Hopkins and H.D. Smith (eds.) *Willard and Spackman's occupational therapy*, 5th edition. Philadelphia: JB Lippincott. 3–23.

Hugman, R. (1991) *Power in caring professions*. Basingstoke: MacMillan.

Hui, A. (2012) Things in motion, things in practice: how mobile practice networks facilitate the travel and use of leisure objects. *Journal of Consumer Culture*, 12(2): 195–215.

Hui, A., Schatzki, T., and Shove, E. (eds.) (2017) *The nexus of practices: connections, constellations, practitioners*. London: Routledge.

Khalsa, S. (n.d.) Elizabeth Blackwell, M.D., America's first female doctor. Amazing women in history. Online at https://amazingwomeninhistory.com/elizabeth-blackwell-first-female-doctor/. Accessed May 2022.

Levin, H. (1938) Occupational and recreational therapy among the ancients. *Occupational Therapy and Rehabilitation*, 17(5): 311–316.

Lidz, T. (1966) Adolph Meyer and the development of American psychiatry. *The American Journal of Psychiatry*, 123(3): 320–332. Reprinted in Serrett, K.D. (ed.) (1985) *Philosophical and historical roots of occupational therapy*. New York: Haworth Press. 33–53.

Low, J.F. (1992) The reconstruction aides. *American Journal of Occupational Therapy*, 46(1): 38–43.

Macdonald, G.L. (1939) The development of occupational therapy in Scotland. *Canadian Journal of Occupational Therapy*, 6(1): 17–20.

Mendez, M.A. (1986) *A chronicle of the World Federation of Occupational Therapists The first thirty years: 1952–1982*. Geneva, Switzerland: WFOT.

Morley, J. (2017) Technologies within and beyond practices. In: A. Hui, T. Schatzki and E. Shove (eds.) *The nexus of practices: connections, constellations, practitioners*. London: Routledge.

Morris, W. (1894) How I became a socialist. Reprinted in Morris, W. (2008) *Useful work versus useless toil*. London: Penguin.

New World Encyclopedia (2020). *Colonialism*. Online at https://www.newworldencyclopedia. org/p/index.php?title=Colonialismandoldid=1033896. Accessed May 2022.

Nicolini, D. (2012) *Practice theory, work and organization: an introduction*. Oxford: Oxford University Press.

Nicolini, D., and Monteiro, P. (2017) The practice approach: for a praxeology of organisational and management studies. In: A. Langley and H. Tsoukas (eds.) *The SAGE handbook of process organization studies*. London: Sage.

O'Sullivan, E. N. M. (1955) *Textbook of occupational therapy: with chief reference to psychological medicine*. London: H. K. Lewis.

Paterson, C.F. (2010) *Opportunities not prescriptions: the development of occupational therapy in Scotland 1900-1960*. Aberdeen: Aberdeen History of Medicine Publications, no. 3.

Reckwitz, A. (2002) Towards a theory of social practices. *European Journal of Social Theory*, 5(2): 243–263.

Reed, K.L., and Sanderson, S.N. (1980) *Concepts of occupational therapy*. Baltimore: Williams and Wilkins.

Reed, K.L., and Sanderson, S.N. (1992) *Concepts of occupational therapy*, 3rd edition. Baltimore: Williams and Wilkins.

Ruskin, J. (1862) *Unto this last*. Reprinted in Cook, E.T. and Wedderburn, A. (eds.) *The works of John Ruskin*, Volume 17. London: George Allen.

Schatzki, T.R. (1996) *Social practices: a Wittgensteinian approach to human activity and the social*. New York: Cambridge University Press.

Schatzki, T.R. (2001) Introduction: practice theory. In: T.R. Schatzki, K. Knorr Cetina and E. von Savigny (eds.) *The practice turn in contemporary social theory*. London: Routledge. 1–14.

Schatzki, T.R. (2002) *The site of the social*. Pennsylvania: Pennsylvania University Press.

Schatzki, T.R. (2010) Materiality and social life. *Nature and Culture*, 5(2): 123–149.

Schatzki, T.R. (2016) Practice theory as a flat ontology. In: G. Spaargaren, D. Weenink and M. Lamers (eds.) *Practice theory and research: exploring the dynamics of social life*. Abingdon: Routledge. 28–42.

Schön, D. (1983) *The reflective practitioner: how professionals thinkin action*. New York: Basic.

Sedlačko, M. (2017) Conducting ethnography with a sensibility for practice. In: M. Jonas, A. Wroblewski and B. Littig (eds.) *Methodological reflections on practice oriented theories*. Springer. 47–60.

Sennett, R. (2008) *The craftsman*. London: Allen Lane.

Serrett, K.D. (1985) Another look at occupational therapy's history: paradigm or pair of hands? In: K.D. Serrett (ed.) *Philosophical and historical roots of occupational therapy*. New York: Haworth Press. 1–31.

Shannon, P.D. (1977) The derailment of occupational therapy. *American Journal of Occupational Therapy*, 31(4): 229–234.

Shove, E., Pantzar, M., and Watson, M. (2012) *The dynamics of social practice: everyday life and how it changes*. London: Sage.

Sivasundaram, S. (2021) *Waves across the south: a new history of revolution and empire*. Chicago: University of Chicago Press.

Social Welfare History Project (2011). Julia Clifford Lathrop (1858–1932): first chief of the children's bureau and advocate for enactment of the Sheppard-Towner maternity and infancy act of 1921. *Social Welfare History Project*. Online at https://socialwelfare.library.vcu.edu/federal/lathrop-julia-clifford/. Accessed May 2022.

Tharoor, S. (2018). *Inglorious empire: what the British did to India*. London: Penguin UK.

Toynbee Hall (n.d.) Our history. Online at www.toynbeehall.org.uk/about-us/our-history. Accessed May 2022.

University of Chicago School of Social Service Administration (n.d). Online at https://www.ssa.uchicago.edu/our-first-century. Accessed May 2022.

von Hoffman, A. (1998) *The origins of American housing reform:* W98-2. Joint Center for Housing Studies. Harvard University.

WFOT (2016) *Minimum standards for the education of occupational therapists: revised 2016*. Online at https://www.wfot.org/resources/new-minimum-standards-for-the-education-of-occupational-therapists-2016-e-copy. Accessed May 25, 2020.

Whipps, J., and Lake, D. (2016) Pragmatist feminism. *Stanford encyclopedia of philosophy*. Online at https://plato.stanford.edu/entries/femapproach-pragmatism/. Accessed May 2022.

Wilcock, A.A. (2001) *Occupation for health, Volume 1: A journey from self health to prescription*. London: British Association and College of Occupational Therapists.

Wilcock, A.A. (2002) *Occupation for health, Volume 2: A journey from prescription to self health*. London: British Association and College of Occupational Therapists.

2 Managerialism and health services

Jennifer Creek

With contributions from Liz Wylde, Jane Clewes, and Rachel Barker

Introduction

As discussed in Chapter 1, occupational therapy came into existence as a discrete entity at the beginning of the 20th century and, along with other healthcare disciplines, followed a process of professionalisation. By the middle of the century, occupational therapy had become, at most, a semi-profession; lacking the power to maintain its position when general management was introduced into health and social care services. Managerialism reduced the power of all the professions, including medicine, and loss of autonomy reduced occupational therapy to more of a technical trade than a profession.

Managerialism and occupational therapy have different, conflicting teleoaffectivities (see glossary): the goal of managerialism is to ensure the overall success of the organisation, in terms of its stability and sustainability, while occupational therapy has always been concerned with providing the most appropriate service to patients and clients. When management has the power to direct what practitioners can and cannot do, all services are provided within the scope of available resources; but occupational therapists may be left with a sense of frustration because they feel that clients are not getting the best possible occupational therapy service. Management prefigures healthcare outcomes by structuring space and time towards the achievement of the goals of the organisation. For example, management shapes occupational therapy outcomes by

- defining the meaning of occupational therapy within the organisation
- controlling what materials are made available
- determining where occupational therapists are allowed to work, such as hospitals and/or clients' homes and workplaces
- specifying the duration of face-to-face sessions and of each client's total intervention
- naming the competences occupational therapists are allowed to use.

This chapter discusses the relationship between occupational therapy and managerialism in three sections. The first section explores what is meant by management and managerialism, and illustrates how a culture of managerialism can come to dominate health services. The second section positions managerialism in relation to neoliberal political and economic ideologies, and considers the role of management in the exercise of power. The third section looks at how managerialism affects the work of occupational therapy practitioners, finishing with a case study to illustrate how one occupational therapist has experienced the impact of general management.

DOI: 10.4324/9781003016755-2

What is managerialism?

This section begins by defining management, scientific management and managerialism. It goes on to describe how an ideology of managerialism can shape the structure and purposes of health services, using the UK National Health Service (NHS) as an illustrative example.

Management

To **manage** means to administer, control and direct the affairs of a state, institution, household or other organisation (Shorter Oxford English Dictionary 2002). **Management** is the action or manner of managing. A **manager** is someone whose role is to direct, supervise, co-ordinate and control the workings of a business or other type of organisation.

Management can be described as a set of social practices that form part of the structure and activity of organisations. It has been suggested 'that practices (in one way or another) are fundamental to the production, reproduction, and transformation of social and organizational matters' (Nicolini 2012: 14). The fundamental reason why an organisation includes management practices is to ensure that it serves its basic purposes, works efficiently, meets its goals, plans ahead, adapts in a controlled way to change and maintains its operations (Richards 2014).

When the workplace for workers is a factory or other organisation, rather than their own homes, the responsibility for controlling and directing work no longer rests with those who produce goods or deliver services but with their managers. This allocation of responsibility also applies to workers in health and social care services, which can be seen as sites for the production of care resources.

In the early 20th century, the idea that management could be a science was initiated in the United States and spread to other industrialised countries. Scientific management is based on four principles, set out by F.W. Taylor in his 1911 book: *The Principles of Scientific Management*.

- Each part of an individual's work is studied and the most efficient method is devised for undertaking each task.
- The most suitable person is chosen to undertake each task, based on competence and motivation. The worker is taught the most efficient way to do the task.
- Managers monitor workers' performance and supervise them to ensure the task is done in the most efficient way.
- There is a clear division of work and responsibility between management and workers. Managers spend their time planning, training and supervising, allowing workers to focus on performing their tasks efficiently (British Library, n.d.).

Scientific management is based on the unscientific assumption that workers are motivated by material rewards and the possibility of advancement, rather than by any sense that work has an intrinsic value. They can, therefore, be directed to undertake any task that the manager allocates to them. One of the unintended consequences of this approach to management is that workers become alienated from their tasks.

Scientific management spread from the United States to other industrialised countries, along with modern methods of production, such as the production line. The person who oversees the operations of an organisation and ensures that it works in the most efficient way is usually called a professional manager or a general manager.

Managerialism

Growing out of scientific management, the ideology of **managerialism** promotes management as the optimal form of directing an organisation and the best way to ensure organisational success (Janse 2019). The second half of the 20th century saw the development of management as a profession, with its own scientific language and specialised techniques (Rose 1989), to the point where it is now widely accepted that professional managers are the best people to direct and control organisations.

Within a culture of managerialism, the work of an organisation is directed by professional managers, not by the workers or the owners. Managers have the power to arrange both the physical environment and the social environment of an organisation. They decide how space is utilised, what equipment is purchased, how the physical environment is organised and what it looks like. In addition, managers decide who can utilise particular spaces and pieces of equipment, who takes responsibility for which parts of the work process and what each person's role is within the organisation at any point in time.

Case study 1 illustrates the process of managerialisation, using the example of the UK National Health Service (NHS).

Case study 1: The managerialisation of healthcare in the United Kingdom

Healthcare services in the United Kingdom were nationalised in 1948, with community health services, primary care and hospitals all becoming part of the newly created NHS (Edwards 1993). Doctors and nurses retained a major role in the management of services, while administrators only had responsibility for managing non-professional staff. Hospitals were managed by teams of three people with equal status: a lay administrator, a senior doctor and the hospital matron.

Concern about the cost of the NHS led to a Committee of Enquiry being set up in 1953, to look at long-term funding issues. The *Guillebaud Report*, which was published in 1956, described the NHS as 'a wealth producing as well as a health producing Service' (Guillebaud et al. 1956) but suggested that there was a need for more supervision and oversight of services.

In 1963, a review was begun of the administration of health services (Edwards 1993), which concluded by recommending a national approach to recruiting, training and developing hospital administrative staff. By the mid-1960s, hospital administrators were responsible for all aspects of the running of hospitals other than clinical services. Despite concerns expressed about variations in the quality of practice, when based on professional judgement (Rivett, n.d.), 'Clinical freedom and independence was fiercely defended by the professions' (Edwards 1993: 14). Throughout the 1960s, there were more calls for organisational reform and clearer lines of responsibility. The *Salmon Report* of 1966 led to the introduction of a management structure for the nursing profession, with ward sisters becoming ward managers and the chief nursing officer reporting to hospital management (Salmon 1966).

In 1967, The Kings Fund published the report of a working party on hospital management, which recommended that the hospital administrator should become the general manager of the hospital, including clinical services (Howard 1967). Many hospital administrators did not have a clinical background and there were tensions between members of the tri-partite hospital management teams, who did not necessarily see the goals of the hospital in the same way. Nonetheless, the King's Fund recommendations were rejected and the idea of management by consensus continued to be popular for some years (Edwards 1993).

During the 1970s, it became government policy to close small hospitals and build large, District General Hospitals that would both concentrate professional expertise and lead to economies of scale. The role of managers became increasingly important in these huge institutions, while professional staff found it 'increasingly difficult to give one-to-one care because of sheer weight of numbers' (Edwards 1993: 46).

Throughout the 1980s, various attempts were made to restructure the NHS so as to increase efficiency and reduce costs. These included the introduction of national performance indicators, external audit and competitive tendering for ancillary services. Then, in 1983, the UK government instituted a 'Management inquiry to give advice on the effective use and management of manpower and related resources in the National Health Service' (Edwards 1993: 79), led by a businessman, Roy Griffiths. *The Griffiths Report*, which was published in October 1983, recommended the introduction of a Health Services Supervisory Board, to be responsible for oversight of the NHS, and a small, multi-disciplinary NHS Management Board, that would 'plan implementation of the policies approved by the Supervisory Board; give leadership to the management of the NHS; control performance; and achieve consistency and drive over the long term' (Griffiths 1983, Recommendation 3). The report called for closer involvement of clinicians in the management process while, at the same time, introducing general management at all levels of the service. One of the functions of general managers was to ensure 'that the professional functions are effectively geared into the overall objectives and responsibilities of the general management process' (op. cit., Observation 9). This was the beginning of a progressive erosion of professional autonomy in making clinical judgements.

In 1989, following another review of the NHS, the government published a white paper, *Working for Patients* (Department of Health 1989). This paper introduced a split between the bodies that provided care, such as hospitals, and those that purchased it, such as District Health Authorities, creating an internal market in the NHS. Henceforth, health authorities would be able to obtain services from NHS hospitals outside their area or from the private sector; as part of their purchasing role, they were expected to consider private providers. The changes set out in the white paper had been fully implemented in England and Wales by 1996 (Levitt et al. 1999: 20).

Working for Patients introduced competition into the NHS, with the argument that it would be a mechanism for improving efficiency. However, it also created the potential for conflict between the financial goals of healthcare organisations and the quality of care given to patients. In pursuit of efficiency and cost savings, work and job roles were reorganised to maximise productivity and worker flexibility, for example, by creating generic care management roles in place of individual professional roles (Whitfield 2006).

Another significant milestone in the managerialisation of the NHS came with the publication of the white paper, *Agenda for Change*, in 1999. This established national pay scales for NHS staff, with two pay spines: one for doctors and dentists and another for non-medical staff. Senior managers had a separate pay structure. The jobs of all non-medical staff, including occupational therapists, were analysed to identify the knowledge and skills required for their performance. The national pay spine had nine bands, each of which was accompanied by a job profile setting out the knowledge and competences expected at that level. One effect of this pay structure was that senior professional staff seeking further promotion had to apply for generic management roles. From 2013, retention of pay level and incremental pay rises were made conditional on locally set performance requirements, and staff became subject to regular performance appraisal.

This section has provided an overview of health service management and the rise of a culture of managerialism in the United Kingdom. The next section describes some of the macro-level impacts of managerialism on healthcare services.

Macro-level issues of managerialism

This section begins with a discussion of neoliberal thinking, how it influences government policy in many countries and how managerialism fits into a neoliberal agenda. This is followed by a brief account of some of the ways in which governments, and other authorities, exercise power to enforce their policies. The section finishes by describing how these issues play out in the management of healthcare services.

Neoliberalism

In the 21st century, economic and political thinking in Western democracies is dominated by neoliberal thought and ideas (Hoggett 2009, Stiglitz 2010). Neoliberal economics are based on the assumption that, if the market is allowed to operate freely, supply and demand will balance each other and there will be enough for everyone. 'An economy structured in the form of relations of exchange between discrete economic units pursuing their undertaking with boldness and energy ... will produce the most social goods and distribute them in the manner most advantageous to each and to all' (Rose 1989: 230). Neoliberalism is, therefore, an approach to governing that favours free-market capitalism, small government, deregulation and reduction in government spending.

Ideally, neoliberal governments step back from regulating the market and allow it to find its own balance. In reality, governments have tended to roll back from intervening in certain areas, such as financial regulation, healthcare, education and social welfare provision, while taking a greater role in other areas, such as internal and external security (Hoggett 2009). When governments draw back from providing public services, these services may be provided in three ways: carried out by individuals and communities, for example, grandparents as unpaid carers for their grandchildren; provided by third sector organisations, such as mental health charities, or taken over by private companies, such as healthcare providers and higher education providers.

Privately provided healthcare services may be financed from general taxation or individual health insurance, the latter often employment-related. Whether private health services are funded by governments or personal insurance, one of their functions is to make profits for their shareholders. A focus on reducing costs to increase profits brings the risk of:

deteriorating working conditions; worse pay, reduced staff levels, greater work-loads, more stress, all of which negatively impact on safety and quality of care. Greater health inequality is fostered as private, for-profit providers 'cherry-pick' lower-risk and paying patients, whilst higher-risk and poorer patients, or those needing emergency care, remain reliant on under-resourced (thanks to austerity) public health service provision.

(Tansey 2017: 1)

In a culture of managerialism, where general managers have the power to direct the work of staff, the success of an organisation may be judged by the profits it makes rather than by other outputs, such as improved population health. For example, government healthcare contracts may be awarded to the company that offers the cheapest services rather than the highest quality of service. This allows the government to contain costs, while responsibility for providing acceptable services within financial constraints is delegated to the private provider.

Governments and organisations use a number of mechanisms to shape people's actions towards the ideals and ends of the organisation. We explore three of these mechanisms of government here: power, rules and authority.

Power, rules and authority

Government is the exercise of authority by one person or group of people over another person or group of people. The term is frequently used to refer to how a country or state is ruled; for example, government by democratically elected representatives or government by a dictator. However, the concept of **governing** can be applied more generally to mean the exercise of power at any scale of society, from the individual to the national level and beyond (Watson 2017).

There are different ways of understanding power but the concept is familiar to everyone and it is indisputably one of the 'constitutive elements of the social reality we experience' (Nicolini 2012: 6). **Power** exists in the relations between people and can be seen as the relative capacity of people within a social system to direct or shape the actions of others. For example, all the members of a family group exercise power over each other to different extents and in different ways, although one person may be dominant.

The dominant person or group within a social system is the one that has the capacity to direct the actions of others and to create or block others' possibilities for action. To the extent that power is a socially constituted, relational effect, it could be viewed as a dimension of inequality, including inequality in capacities, resources or autonomy.

Whether at the level of the individual, the social group or the nation, power is exercised and its effects are experienced through a variety of means. **Rules**, for example, are social mechanisms for directing people to perform specific actions in particular ways (Schatzki 2010), such as which side of the road motorists must drive on. Some rules are formalised into procedures, laws or protocols but many are experienced as social norms or standards of conduct (Watson 2017), such as the acceptable distance to be maintained between people in different cultures and social situations.

Within any social group, some people are in a stronger position than others to direct the actions of members of the group: they have authority. **Authority** is a social position that confers power to enforce obedience or to influence action (Shorter Oxford English Dictionary 2002). Authority may derive from knowledge: for example, the university lecturer has authority over students by virtue of knowing more than they do about the subject being studied. It may also be held by force, as when the military of a country seizes power from the elected government. Authority may also come with possession of resources, which brings the power to decide how those resources are allocated, such as a landowner deciding the purposes for which the land is used.

Authority is exercised through certain actions being approved, authorised or re- quired while others are prohibited, disapproved or illegal. Sanctioned actions are rewarded by the social group, such as paying people for productive work, while non- sanctioned actions are punished, such as meting out prison sentences for certain types of theft.

There is a tendency for those with power, the social elites, to use their influence to retain and extend their power; directing people's actions to maintain social order and thereby producing and reproducing differences and inequalities (Nicolini 2012). Thus, structures of privilege and advantage become systematised across space and time through the performance of social practices. However, the dynamic nature of social structures means they are always open to contestation, as members of the social group strive to take more power for themselves through their actions.

The next section investigates how these mechanisms of government play out in the management of healthcare services.

Management of healthcare services

The way that healthcare services are provided by governments is strongly influenced by how health is conceptualised. For example, if health is seen as a property of communities or as a human right, there will be a strong focus on public health; on tackling the causes of disease and promoting good health in populations. If health is seen as a personal quality or individual responsibility, the focus will be on providing goods and services that individuals can use to protect their health, such as sports clubs, or that treat disease, such as medicinal drugs.

Neoliberal governments view health as a necessary constituent of a competitive labour force, in the context of a global marketplace: healthy workers are more pro- ductive than workers who take time off work due to sickness. They also see health as an individual responsibility; a responsibility that would be undermined by the pro- vision of universal, low-cost healthcare services. In order to provide the most efficient and effective healthcare, these governments apply the logic of the market to health services, on the assumption that competition and deregulation will result in more health for less money (Hoggett 2009). Some areas of healthcare need, such as older people, those with long-term conditions and people with learning disabilities, areas in which occupational therapists have traditionally worked, are unlikely to contribute to the economy and therefore do not attract funding. Furthermore, a free-market economy requires continual growth. Health service managers have to think not just about making things work in the present but also about expansion and where the next contract is coming from. The current service has to be just good enough for the or- ganisation to keep winning contracts.

When healthcare services are seen as businesses, in competition with other busi- nesses for both resources and contracts, conflict can arise between the practices of managers and those of front-line staff, as the two groups are driven by different tel-eoaffectivities. The remit of the general manager is to produce the most health for the least expenditure, by continually reducing costs and increasing the productivity of the organisation; while front-line staff want to achieve the highest possible level of care for each person they see. Additionally, the different professions have to compete with each other for limited resources by balancing results against costs. This can lead to more attention being paid to the people who are more likely to recover quickly rather than those who need long-term care or rehabilitation.

In the previous section, authority was defined as a social position that confers power to enforce obedience or to influence action. It is usual for the general managers of health services to have authority over all aspects of the organisation, including clinical services. This means that they can direct the performance of the service towards meeting management goals rather than clinical goals. An example of this is given in Box 2.1.

Box 2.1   Conflict of interest

An occupational therapist was interviewing a man in the accident and emergency department (A&E) of the hospital. He was disclosing some highly personal and sensitive information when the curtain was suddenly swished back by A&E staff, who said that the patient would have to move down the corridor to the next section. The hospital contract specified that each patient would be dealt with within three hours, and this man had now reached that limit. If he was not moved, A&E would be fined for breaching the target. Although the man was fully mobile, he had to get back onto a trolley and wait for a porter to wheel him down the corridor, because the occupational therapist was not allowed to do this.

This major interruption to the occupational therapist's intervention, due to procedures and targets set by management, had a negative impact on the quality of care given to the client. The mental health liaison team manager had made several requests for a private interview room to be created in A&E for the team to use but, since liaison services were not directly employed by the hospital, management wanted to charge a fee for the rent of a room.

Health service managers exercise power through mechanisms such as the replacement of professional expertise and judgement with standardised procedures, checklists, guidelines and protocols. Matthew Crawford, an American political philosopher, linked the rise of managerialism with a progressive separation of knowledge from its practical application: 'scattered craft knowledge is concentrated in the hands of the employer, then doled out again to workers in the form of minute instructions needed to perform some *part* of what is now a work *process*' (Crawford 2009: 39). What the healthcare worker does is determined not by their professional reasoning but by standardised procedures that have been agreed at management level, reducing professional practice to a series of technical tasks. Under this system, a worker's ability to do the assigned job is judged not on the outcomes but on her or his 'capability to complete a series of independent tasks of varying complexity in a standardised manner' (Maxwell and Leary 2020: 1). The problem with adopting this approach for dealing with complex problems is that the performance of healthcare workers is only assessed against a specified set of competences and not against 'the need to balance competing tasks, or to consider the unintended consequences of one task on another aspect of the workload' (Maxwell and Leary 2020: 1). An example of such unintended consequences is given in Box 2.2.

Box 2.2   Task competence without professional judgement

A man was admitted to the hospital following a major stroke. A nurse was stationed by his bed to lift his affected leg back onto the mattress whenever it slipped off: the nurse had been instructed just to do this one task. The contractors who provided domestic and catering services regularly refreshed the man's water jug, as specified in the service contract, which was on a table at the foot of his bed. The man was becoming more confused so he was referred to the mental health liaison service and visited by an occupational therapist.

When the occupational therapist assessed the man's mental state, he thought that he was back in the pit (he had been a coal miner); he was unable to co-ordinate his hand and eyes to grasp an object held out to him; he could not say whether he was thirsty, when he last had a drink or whether there was drinking water available. It was evident that he was seriously dehydrated, despite having full-time, individual nursing care. Further investigation showed that the man had sustained a hospital-acquired, acute kidney injury on top of chronic kidney disease; he now needed intra-venous rehydration.

Healthcare organisations not only have to provide the services specified in contracts, to an agreed standard, but also have to record evidence that this has been done. The focus is on meeting targets and carrying out agreed numbers of procedures rather than on health outcomes, which can be harder to measure. The requirement to measure and record what has been done has resulted in 'the development of a vast array of inspectorates and performance management systems' (Hoggett 2009); such as performance indicators, internal and external audit, performance monitoring, quality control and risk management. Many of these systems require front-line staff to record, in minute detail, their activities throughout the working day, taking time that might otherwise have been spent in-patient care.

These performance monitoring systems have several weaknesses; for example, they only measure what can be quantified, such as number of patients seen, length of time in hospital and percentage of mandatory training undertaken by staff. Aspects of care that are more challenging to measure, such as actively listening to the patient and treating people with respect, are ignored. It has been suggested that having to do what can be recorded, rather than doing the right thing, has encouraged the creation of a virtual reality; an auditable surface of statistics, reports and reviews that then gets confused with the reality it represents (Hoggett 2009). An example of this is given in Box 2.3.

Box 2.3 Following procedure

Jane took her exhausted, weak and poorly father to A&E, where he was put on a hydrating drip and eventually got to sleep. The standard procedure in A&E was to take each patient's blood pressure every two hours. When Jane asked why staff were waking her father regularly to take his blood pressure, she was told that it was standard procedure. She then asked what would be done if her father's blood pressure was found to be high or low and was told that no action would be taken. Jane asked what staff were doing when they woke her father to take his blood pressure; their response was that they were monitoring it.

The future of healthcare services is prefigured by the social practices, material arrangements and teleoaffective structures that constitute those services in the present. **Prefiguration** refers to the way that possible courses of action are qualified, by the arrangement of the social context, 'on such registers as easy and hard, obvious and obscure, tiresome and invigorating, short and long, and so on' (Schatzki 2010: 140). In other words, the arrangement of healthcare practices and possible patterns of population health in the future are qualified by the relevant practices, material arrangements and teleoffective structures of any given present. Possible future levels of population health are both expanded and limited by the social present; that is, by the form of present healthcare and public health practices (such as the relative resourcing of primary and secondary healthcare), the material arrangements that are sustained by those practices (such as the places where healthcare can be accessed), the obduracy of material structures that supported previous practices (such as old hospital buildings) and teleoaffective structures (such as neoliberal values and categorisations of illness).

This section has discussed some of the mechanisms by which those in power influence and constrain the practices of workers; specifically how healthcare management controls the work of professional staff. The next section explores how these mechanisms work in practice, using a case study to illustrate how they are experienced by an occupational therapy practitioner.

Micro-level issues of managerialism

The macro understanding and organisation of healthcare in a managerialised world, as described above, affect how practitioners see their role and function and also what they do. This section explores the impact of management on the day-to-day practice of occupational therapy, followed by a case study to illustrate how that impact is experienced by one practitioner.

The work of an organisation is carried out through the performance of a range of different practices within the context of that organisation; such as management, production, administration and marketing. The ways in which all these practices are performed are strongly influenced by the arrangement of physical and social conditions within that context. 'The arrangement of a context for certain practices gives significance to certain possibilities, activities, purposes and concerns while others are left out or made difficult to pursue' (Dreier 2008: 32). For example, during the COVID-19 pandemic of 2020, many routine interventions were cancelled, by hospitals in the United Kingdom and elsewhere, in order to make space, time and other resources available for treating people whose lives were threatened by the infection.

In practice theory, the physical and social arrangement of a context is said to prefigure the scope of possibilities for action within that context. In an organisation that has espoused the ideology of managerialism, it is managers who have the greatest power, through the ordering of physical and social systems and structures, to prefigure the scope of possibilities for the action of all the workers within that organisation. For example, the general manager of a mental health hospital decides to close the occupational therapy department and convert the space into a mother and baby unit. This decision opens up new possibilities for mothers with mental health problems to bring their babies into the hospital with them, thus avoiding a break in their motherhood practices. At the same time, it limits the possibility of occupational therapy practice taking place within the hospital boundaries but away from the wards. Thus, management decisions can sometimes prefigure the context in ways that leave the occupational therapist less scope for flexibility and improvisation.

Case study 1 offered an example of how a culture of managerialism in UK health services has shifted the balance of power from medical, nursing and other front-line professions to general managers, making it possible for management practices to take precedence over clinical practices. This shift is experienced by healthcare practitioners in a number of ways, including proceduralisation, de-professionalisation, performance monitoring and sanctions.

Proceduralisation

General management of healthcare services is not concerned with individual patients but with 'the achievement of plans through tasks and processes' (Barr 2008: 167). Managers set goals for the healthcare organisation and require employees to embrace those goals. To ensure compliance from healthcare staff, managers may also specify the processes that should be followed to reach those goals; in the form of, for example, protocols for designated areas of practice, care pathways for well-defined groups of patients and guidelines to support clinical decision-making. Each of these tools delimits what the clinician can and cannot do, thus reducing the professional autonomy of practitioners to select the actions they judge most appropriate to take in particular circumstances. The style of management that requires workers to follow standard procedures is based on a behaviour-oriented contract between the organisation and the professional, in which the focus of the service is on process rather than outcomes (Eisenhardt 1989).

When interventions are manualised as sets of tasks to be performed in specified circumstances, occupational therapists may come to mistake the general aim of their role with the list of tasks they have been apportioned. Concerns about following protocols, keeping within the rules and not contravening management-defined boundaries can lead to staff failing to see what the client's real needs are. This was illustrated in Box 2.3, when nursing staff kept waking an exhausted patient to take his blood pressure because it was standard procedure.

De-professionalisation

One of the roles of the health service manager is to 'allocat[e] front-line resources in a manner which [will] exact more from workers for less' (Worth 2018: 6). To achieve this, the principles of scientific management are applied to professional staff as well as to ancillary workers. The result is an undermining of professionalism, as 'the cognitive elements of the job are appropriated from professionals, instantiated in a system or process, and then handed back to a new class of workers ... who replace the professionals' (Crawford 2009: 44). For example, an occupational therapist working on a forensic mental health ward is expected to assess patients, set goals with them and plan their treatment programmes. Treatment activities are then carried out by therapy assistants.

The reduction of professional roles to lists of tasks allows for generic working, which means that aspects of care are not the domain of particular professions but can be carried out by any person with the appropriate competences. While this system increases workforce flexibility, it can also lead to devaluing of professional skills and even, over time, to loss of profession-specific skills, as the time for teaching and practising them is given over to generic working (Reeves and Summerfield-Mann 2004). An expectation that all staff will be competent to carry out a wide range of generic tasks means that occupational therapists have to devote some of their continuing professional development time to developing generic competences, sometimes at the expense of their profession-specific development. For example, if the running of activity groups is delegated to support staff (see Case study 2), the occupational therapist will not only fail to develop expertise in leading groups but is unlikely to be supported to undertake additional training in that area of practice.

Performance monitoring

To ensure that workers follow specified procedures, demonstrate the required competences for their role and meet targets set by the organisation, managers use various tools for monitoring staff performance. Workers are expected to collect and record data; such as, whether they have met their targets, how their time is used throughout the day and the duration of programmes of intervention (see Case study 2). This is in addition to the records they keep about the clients they are working with. Records are also kept of when staff complete their mandatory training and how much sick leave they take.

The performance of occupational therapy practitioners is monitored through supervision and appraisal systems. Clinical staff are expected to receive regular supervision from a more senior professional in order to check that they are coping with their work, to provide a forum for discussing challenging cases and to give support. The annual appraisal, which is done by a senior manager, involves two-way feedback about the practitioner's performance and is an opportunity to identify training or other development needs.

Sanctions

Management ensures compliance from healthcare workers: first, by determining the competences they should have, setting out the procedures to be followed in each case and specifying the standards of performance to be achieved; and, then, by measuring their performance and applying sanctions if it falls short. The introduction of standardised packages of care for staff to use with their patients makes it easier to measure and record performance by eliminating skills that are hard to measure, for example, professional reasoning and judgement. If staff do not follow standardised procedures, or fall short of the required standard of performance, or fail to meet the targets set by managers, they may be subject to a range of sanctions, including not receiving a pay increment, being subject to increased supervision or having their contract of employment terminated.

In times of economic austerity, job opportunities and choices become more limited and there is pressure to conform to the requirements of employing authorities or risk redundancy. In some countries, such as the United States, health insurance is an employer benefit so that staff risk losing health cover as well as their salary, if they leave their job, increasing the pressure to conform.

The following case study provides an illustration of how management is experienced by an occupational therapist working for the UK NHS.

Case study 2: The impact of management on the occupational therapist. By Elizabeth Wylde

Kimberley is an occupational therapist working in a specialist autism service. This service is for autistic adults who do not have a learning disability or complex mental health needs. The autism team provide three key services: diagnostic assessment of autism; support for autistic adults and their siblings, partners or parents, and professional consultation and training for those working with autistic individuals. The service is based in a small hospital, which has some in-patient wards and also hosts a variety of community teams and outpatient departments. The autism department is set in a converted ward, with space for offices as well as clinic rooms. The service covers three local authority areas, which include a city, four large towns and several villages in outlying rural areas. Anyone can refer to the service, whether they are seeking diagnostic assessment or seeking support. Typically, although the service does receive referrals from GPs and other professionals, the majority are self-referrals.

The service is funded by the national government and hosted by the local health board but is integrated with the three local authorities. The service manager and clinicians in the team are employed by the NHS, which has its own pay scales and conditions of employment, while support staff are employed by the three local authorities, under different terms and conditions. The team is made up of three groups of staff:

- support and administrative staff, who are employed at a salary equivalent to NHS pay band 3
- clinicians, who are employed at NHS pay band 7
- management, which consists of a clinical lead employed at NHS pay band 8b and a service manager employed at NHS pay band 8a.

Kimberley is managed on a day-to-day basis by the service manager, who reports to the locality lead for mental health and, from there, the chain of command continues up until it reaches the health board chief executive. However, the Strategic Lead of

Occupational Therapy for Mental Health within the health board also holds line management responsibility for Kimberley and provides her with clinical supervision. Kimberley receives further clinical supervision, on the generic aspects of her role, from the team clinical lead, who has no management responsibility for her.

There is a requirement from senior management and the executive team that services record statistics about their performance. Departments are rated on scorecards, which record such figures as waiting list times, number of people on the waiting list, length of time from first appointment to discharge, staff sickness levels and compliance with mandatory training. These data are purely business-focused: data on service user satisfaction is recorded and collated by the National Autism Team, which is funded by the national government and hosted by the Local Government Association, working in partnership with Public Health. For the service manager and the service team, there is a fine balance between meeting targets and producing favourable statistics versus providing a good service that meets the needs of the autistic population.

Kimberley's role in the team includes: carrying out diagnostic assessments, occupational therapy assessments and occupational therapy interventions; providing clinical supervision to support staff; offering professional consultation and training staff. Another important element of Kimberley's role is identifying training opportunities for support staff and helping them to develop in their roles. She also works collaboratively with the clinical lead to help develop the service as a whole. In all these roles, management impacts Kimberley in a multitude of ways; some positive, such as personal development, and some negative, such as frustration at being limited by service constraints.

Having two managers can be confusing and uncomfortable for Kimberley. For example, there is an expectation for her to report to both the service manager and the head of occupational therapy for sickness, annual leave, mandatory training and the annual appraisal. There are additional expectations from the occupational therapy manager, such as a requirement to offer student placements and to attend a quarterly occupational therapy meeting. There are also expectations from the service manager for Kimberley to: attend weekly MDT and team meetings, meet targets, such as her diagnostic assessment quota, and clinically supervise support staff. There can be a lot of demands placed on Kimberley and on her time, and there have been occasions when a conflict of priorities has had to be carefully managed and negotiated by Kimberley. However, the two managers have good lines of communication between them and Kimberley is generally included in that communication, often by email or through regular, three-way supervision. Both managers support Kimberley to set goals for both personal and service development.

The service manager has supported Kimberley to develop in both her leadership and clinical roles. Although there have sometimes been difficult conversations, these have always been followed with actions and points for learning, which have ultimately given Kimberley opportunities to develop skills in delegating, working flexibly, particularly during times where the team is under pressure, and being assertive, especially when trying to challenge the status quo and bring about change. The service manager is well aware of Kimberley's clinical strengths in diagnostic assessment and occupational therapy. Kimberley has been able to demonstrate how occupational therapy makes a tangible difference to the lives of autistic adults and this is recognised and appreciated by the service manager. As a result, the occupational therapy part of her role is, to some extent, protected.

Despite the good working relationships between Kimberley and her managers, there is a conflict of priorities. With relentless demands from executives and senior management for favourable statistics, particularly in relation to waiting times, there is pressure on Kimberley to carry out more diagnostic work to address the significant waiting list, resulting in reduced opportunities to offer occupational therapy sessions. This is frustrating for Kimberley, as it means there is little time to see individuals beyond the assessment phase. As a result, the occupational therapy role has become more consultative, often involving offering solutions that involve supporting staff rather than delivering direct occupational therapy interventions. There is an expectation from management that interventions are time-limited and make the most efficient use of resources therefore when occupational therapy intervention is required, this is generally for brief interventions. Kimberley will often complete the initial assessment and formulate a plan with the individual, then pass the person on to support staff to carry out the intervention.

Although this division of labour may appear more efficient to management, seeming to free up Kimberley's time for diagnostic and occupational therapy assessments, it can be costly in different ways. Interventions carried out by support staff may take longer, as they need regular supervision and support throughout the intervention; a process that ultimately takes up more of both the support workers' and Kimberley's time. From Kimberley's perspective, there is a real sense of frustration. Although she may carry out the assessment, goal setting and intervention planning, Kimberley misses working alongside people to see them grow and achieve their goals. Kimberley often finds herself wondering how an individual is progressing: she craves the feedback and evaluation that are key parts of the occupational therapy process and that would let her know if her assessment was valid. Also, it can feel uncomfortable for Kimberley and the autistic individual to part ways early on in the intervention process; both parties have worked to develop a rapport. When the sessions end the person has to develop that rapport with someone new.

Personality and management style have a clear impact on team morale and productivity. A rigid adherence to hierarchy can be frustrating for staff at lower levels, although this can work in their favour when senior staff in the team act as a buffer for the downward pressure from senior management. However, there are times when issues filter through to all members of the team, particularly if mistakes have been made. The senior manager's preferred method of contact with clinical staff is to highlight mistakes by sending group emails. This style of communication can be demoralising for Kimberley and other staff members, leaving them feeling uneasy and wondering who made the mistake. On the other hand, the service manager is keen to promote and support well-being in the team; good work is often highlighted and praised, and time and space are made available to ensure staff take adequate breaks.

Overall, for Kimberley, there is a feeling of instability in her work role. At times, this is manageable; she can adapt to change and cope with the pressures. However, sometimes it does not feel manageable and can lead to thoughts of leaving the service.

Summary and conclusion

This chapter began by explaining the concepts of management and managerialism. A case study, describing the progressive managerialisation of the UK National Health Service, was used to illustrate the impact a culture of managerialism can have on the way health services are organised and delivered.

The second section linked the rise of managerialism in the 20th century to the neoliberal ideology that dominates economic and political thinking in Western democracies. A description was given of some of the mechanisms through which organisations control the actions of workers, shaping them towards the achievement of the organisation's goals. The section finished with some examples of how health service management operates to align working practices with neoliberal values and goals.

The third section focussed on occupational therapy practice and how it can be facilitated or constrained by the management practices of organisations where occupational therapists work. The impact of managerialism on the day-to-day practice of occupational therapists operates through four instruments of control: proceduralisation, de-professionalisation, performance monitoring and sanctions. A case study was used to explore how one occupational therapy practitioner experiences the positive and negative effects of working in a managerialised service.

The aim of this book is to support occupational therapy practitioners as they navigate the systems within which or through which they work. It does this by identifying occupational therapy as a constellation of social practices, functioning within a wider social context. The deeper our understanding of social context in which occupational therapy operates, the more able we are to work out effective strategies for carrying out our professional purpose. This chapter and the previous one considered the broader historical and political contexts of occupational therapy's development, from its origins at the beginning of the 20th century to its current position and status. The next two chapters explore in more depth how the professional purpose and performance of occupational therapy play out in space and time.

References

Barr, L. (2008) Management. In: J. Creek and L. Lougher (eds.) *Occupational therapy and mental health,* 4th ed. Edinburgh: Churchill Livingstone Elsevier. 159–171.

British Library (n.d.) *Frederick Winslow Taylor.* Online at https://www.bl.uk/people/frederick-winslow-taylor. Accessed May 2022.

Crawford, M.B. (2009) *Shop class as soulcraft: an inquiry into the value of work.* New York: Penguin.

Department of Health (1989) *Working for patients.* London: HMSO.

Dreier, O. (2008) *Psychotherapy in everyday life.* Cambridge: Cambridge University Press.

Edwards, B. (1993) *The National Health Service: a manager's tale 1946-1992.* London: Nuffield Provincial Hospitals Trust. Online at www.nuffieldtrust.org.uk/files/2017-01/a-managers-tale-web-final.pdf. Accessed May 2021.

Eisenhardt, K.M. (1989) Agency theory: an assessment and review. *Academy of Management Review,* 14(1): 57–74.

Griffiths. E.R. (1983) *NHS management inquiry: Griffiths report on NHS October 1983.* Online at www.sochealth.co.uk/national-health-service/griffiths-report-october-1983/. Accessed May 2021.

Guillebaud, C.W., Cook, J.W., Godwin, B.A., Maude, J., and Vickers G. (1956) *Report of the Committee of Enquiry into the Cost of the National Health Service.* Cmd. 9663.

Hoggett, P. (2009) *Politics, identity and emotion.* Boulder, CO: Paradigm.

Howard, G.P.E. (1967) *The shape of hospital management in 1980?: the report of a Joint Working Party set up by the King's Fund and the Institute of Hospital Administrators to consider the future pattern of management in hospitals with particular reference to the needs of district hospitals.* London: King Edward's Hospital Fund for London.

Janse, B. (2019). Managerialism theory. Online at https://www.toolshero.com/management/managerialism-theory/. Accessed May 2022.

Levitt, R., Wall, A., and Appleby, J. (1999) *The reorganized national health service,* 6th ed. Cheltenham: Stanley Thornes. https://core.ac.uk/download/pdf/29943586.pdf

Maxwell, E., and Leary, A. (2020) In praise of professional judgement. *British Medical Journal.* Online at https://blogs.bmj.com/bmj/2020/05/26/elaine-maxwell-alison-leary-praise-professional-judgment/. Accessed May 2022.

Nicolini, D. (2012) *Practice theory, work, and organization: an introduction.* Oxford: Oxford University Press.

Reeves, S., and Summerfield-Mann, L. (2004) Overcoming problems with generic working for occupational therapists based in community mental health settings. *British Journal of Occupational Therapy*, 67(6): 265–268. 10.1177/030802260406700605

Richards, G. (2014) Management and leadership. In: W. Bryant, J. Fieldhouse and K. Bannigan (eds.) *Creek's occupational therapy and mental health*, 5th ed. Edinburgh: Churchill Livingstone Elsevier. 120–131.

Rivett,G. (n.d.) *The history of the National Health Service.* Nuffield Trust. Online at https://www.nuffieldtrust.org.uk/chapter/1968–1977-rethinking-the-national-health-service-1. Accessed February 2022.

Rose, N. (1989) *Governing the soul: the shaping of the private self,* 2nd ed. London: Free Association Books.

Salmon, B. (1966) *Report of the Committee on Senior Nurse Staffing Structure.* London: HMSO.

Schatzki, T.R. (2010) *The timespace of human activity: on performance, society, and history as indeterminate teleological events.* Lanham: Lexicon Books.

Shorter Oxford English Dictionary (2002) *Shorter Oxford English Dictionary on historical principles*, 5th edition. Oxford: Oxford University Press.

Stiglitz, J. (2010) In praise of pluralism. In: D. Ransom and V. Baird (eds.) *People first economics*. Oxford: New Internationalist. 37–46.

Tansey, R. (2017) *The creeping privatisation of healthcare: problematic EU policies and the corporate lobby push.* Corporate European Observatory. Online at https://corporateeurope.org/en/power-lobbies/2017/06/creeping-privatisation-healthcare. Accessed May 2022.

Watson, M. (2017) Placing power in practice theory. In: A. Hui, T. Schatzki , and E. Shove (eds) *The nexus of practices: connections, constellations, practitioners.* London: Routledge.

Whitfield, D. (2006) *A typology of privatisation and marketisation.* European Services Strategy Unit. Online at www.european-services-strategy.org.uk. Accessed May 2022.

Worth, E. (2018) A tale of female liberation? The long shadow of de-professionalization on the lives of post-war women. Revue Francaise de Civilisation Britannique, XXIII-1. http://journals.openedition.org/rfcb/1778

3 Space-time, temporality and professional roles

Kate Sherry, Jennifer Creek, and Michael Allen

Introduction

Practice theory holds that social life, including the practice of professions, is made up of social practices. A practice can be as small as answering the telephone or as large as practising occupational therapy. Conceptualising occupational therapy as a social practice allows us not only to focus on the small and large doings and sayings that constitute the profession but also to identify those doings and sayings as part of a wider social context. This approach to theorising can help us to understand how occupational therapy connects with, contributes to and is shaped by the social life of the communities within which it is practised.

When we are thinking about our work as occupational therapists, it is useful to consider a number of dimensions. In this chapter and the next one, the focus is on the professional purpose and performance of occupational therapy in space-time. While space and time cannot be treated separately, the emphasis in this chapter is on occupational therapy unfolding through time as a social practice, both entity and performance. In Chapter 4, more attention is given to the spatial aspects of occupational therapy in space-time.

As discussed in Chapter 1, examining our work through a practice theory lens reveals that what occupational therapists do takes on different meanings depending on the specific time and space of which it is a part. We see that doing occupational therapy cannot be reduced to repetitions of specific procedures, independent of the spatial-temporal context, on the basis that 'this is how we do it'. We may be tempted to think that occupational therapy practice can be limited to a set of pre-determined steps, especially where the role of the occupational therapist is unclear or confusing, or for students and inexperienced therapists. However, this approach does not take into account the complexity of effective practice. As occupational therapy is introduced and developed in different countries, cultures, settings, time periods and situations, and as realities change over time in settings where the profession is well established, we have to reconsider what we do as occupational therapists, and what our doing might mean in the particular context where we are practising, both in space (physical, social, cultural and political) and in time. We need to think about where the profession is going, in the small practices we perform every day as well as in the larger issues of where we work and who pays us.

In this chapter, time is discussed as a feature of practice and a focus for professional reasoning. The first section explores practice theory conceptualisations of time and briefly introduces its relation to space (which is the topic of the next

DOI: 10.4324/9781003016755-3

chapter). The second section considers time in relation to how occupational therapy roles may be structured; that is, how time is 'spent' and 'managed', and who makes these decisions. The status of occupational therapy as a profession is discussed, with reference to Chapters 1 and 2. The third section of the chapter explores time in day-to-day occupational therapy practice, using a case study from rural South Africa to illustrate professional reasoning around temporal dimensions of service provision and design.

Space-time

Time and space do not exist as separate entities but as a single space-time. In this section, the two terms are first defined and discussed separately, in order to acknowledge that there are different ways of conceptualising them, and then as a unified entity.

What is time?

There are many ways of understanding the phenomenon of time. **Objective time** is not relative to anything external to itself. It is the flow and pace of events that can be measured by the ticking of a clock (the so-called clock time) or the oscillation frequency of caesium atoms (as in atomic clocks) (Encyclopedia Britannica 2021). It is a concept that allows us to think about such matters as: when things happen; how long they happen for; whether other things are happening simultaneously or sequentially; what order things happen in and so on. However, according to Adam (1990), while time must be considered a fact of life, to treat objective time as though it were concrete reality is to obscure and diminish the roles of other conceptualisations of time that are important for understanding the social world. This is because time is also perceived subjectively.

Lived time is a variable aspect of everyday life that is derived from subjective experiences of the social world. Time sometimes seems to go slowly while, at other times, it hurries past, leaving us to wonder where it went. People can feel time-squeezed, pressed for time or harried (Southerton and Tomlinson 2005). Weekends might be perceived differently from weekdays because of the different activities that happen on those days (Shove 2009). There are breakfast times, lunchtimes and dinnertimes, each with its own temporal conventions, such as eating breakfast in the morning or eating soup before the main course and the main course before dessert in a three-course dinner (Shove 2009). A person's attitude towards time-keeping might lead others to think of them as punctual, tardy, lazy or laid back. Depending on the cultural context, someone can be stereotyped according to their personal circadian rhythm, for example, as a night owl, or their time of life, for example, a living national treasure. Such stereotypes may be positive, negative or neutral. Subjective perceptions and understandings of the temporal aspects of daily life have important implications for how our personal, social and work lives are organised and carried on.

Both objective time and subjective, lived time are relevant when thinking about social practices, including occupational therapy. Occupational therapists need an understanding of time as experienced by their clients in order to understand their clients' occupations in context, but also to understand their own practices and the implications of their actions.

Consideration of objective time highlights how practices compete for time as a finite resource; time spent performing one practice is inevitably not available for the performance of other practices. For example, when an occupational therapist takes on the role of manager or care coordinator there is less time available for practising occupational therapy. Objective time also reveals how practice performances are scheduled and sequenced. It shows how practices persist through time as entities, even when they are not being performed; and how they evolve or cease to be, as practice elements combine and recombine in different configurations, endure periods of dormancy or cease to combine in such a way as to be recognisable as a particular practice (Shove, Pantzar and Watson 2012).

The ends to which human activities are oriented are part of teleoaffective structures of practices (see Chapter 1). Teleoaffective structures are 'array[s] of ends, projects, uses (of things), and even emotions that are acceptable or prescribed for participants in [a] practice' (Schatzki 2005: 471–472). From this perspective, we can see that time, as experienced through human activity, is not a characteristic of the individual but of the practice. Different practices have different teleoaffective structures that can be incompatible and compete for the time and resources of practitioners, as in the above example of an occupational therapist practising as a manager or care coordinator. Pursuing the ends of one practice can make pursuing the ends of another practice difficult or even impossible.

Furthermore, no conceptualisations of time are universal but are all strongly influenced by cultural beliefs and values.

Cultural understandings of time

Understandings of time vary across cultures in ways that affect how activities and practices are performed, as well as affecting the relationships between practices, including their timing, sequence and even whether certain practices are performed at all. Where different cultural understandings of time come together, as when an occupational therapist is working with first-generation immigrants, these understandings can come into conflict. Some examples are given here of different cultural conceptualisations of time.

The Native American Hopi are one of several peoples around the world whose language does not conceptualise time as an objective reality (see Tuan 1977; Adam 1990; Loy 2001). Applying only an objective conception of time would impede attempts to understand Hopi culture and practices. For example, the Hopi have no way of expressing, in their language, that it is a hot summer because, linguistically, the concepts of hot and summer have an inextricable association (Loy 2001). Working with groups that have diverse understandings of time has consequences that go beyond the exploration of culture to affect occupational therapy practice.

Many African cultures place particular values on the use of time. In traditional settings, African time is characterised by a leisurely approach to carrying out planned activities, with little effort to control events and an absence of urgency based on perceived time scarcity. In many African communities, taking time with people is a way of communicating the value placed on the relationship, which has primacy over any task or goal one has to achieve. This can mean leisurely greeting processes, long pauses and time spent sitting in companionable silence before the business of a visit or meeting is broached. To be in a hurry with one's agenda is perceived as rude and even suspicious. To a professional used to Western values around not wasting time (one's own or other people's), this can feel uncomfortable. The significance of the communication style may be entirely missed. By holding a typical professional focus on spoken words and active content in an encounter (what is done and what is said), one may miss that others are tuned into something very different (how it is done and who says it) (Sherry et al. 2020).

Another example of how conflicting cultural understandings of time can affect people on a practical level comes from Australia. Prior to colonisation, the Wiradjuri people had no abstract conception of time; time was rather seen in terms of events (Yalmambirra 2000). Hunting and gathering happened when they became necessary; eating happened when hunger set in, and sleeping and waking occurred in accordance with solar rhythms rather than at prescribed times. Consequently, 'Wiradjuri people's life was not regulated by time, as you know time to be' (Yalmambirra 2000: 134). During the early 20th century, Australian government policy attempted to enforce Western values as a means of managing what was perceived as 'an aboriginal problem'. Aboriginal children, including the Wiradjuri, were forced into boarding schools, where those who failed to adhere to the strict routines and schedules that aligned with occidental clock time suffered terrible physical abuse (Yalmambirra 2000). Such policies, imposing Western notions by force, have had devastating consequences for indigenous peoples across the globe (George et al. 2019). The destruction of traditional culture, ways of life, and social fabric has had long-lasting psychosocial impacts. In Canada, for example, Inuit adolescents continue to have an unusually high suicide rate (Tan 2021), and substance abuse is rife amongst American and Australian First Nations people (Benner et al. 2018; George et al. 2019; Purcell-Khodr et al. 2020).

Making sense of these events requires an awareness of how the conflict between cultural understandings of time (in the Australian example, a dominant Western clock time and a subjugated Wiradjuri time) unfolds as part of social practices, with real and sometimes devastating consequences.

What is space?

As with time, there are multiple ways of understanding the phenomenon of space. **Objective space** is intuitively understood as a three-dimensional container bounded by height, width and depth. The notion of objective space assumes that space is a fundamental quantity that provides a framework within which events take place. Whilst it is useful to have absolute quantities of length, height, depth and so on, with which to measure certain aspects of human activity, such approaches can lead to misapprehension of how the human world is constructed. The concept of **relative space** refers to the understanding that space is affected by what takes place within it (Massey 1999). Introducing the concept of relative space inevitably leads to time being included in considerations of space: if space is affected by what occurs within it, it can no longer be separated from the time taken for events to occur.

The idea of a unified space-time is returned to in Chapter 4; here, it is useful to point to two problems for the study of the human world posed by the concept of absolute space. First, the separation of space from time negates the dynamic quality of the events that take place in a given space. This misrepresents human life as static, or reducible to a mapped existence, which yields no information about what human beings actually do in particular spaces. As Bollnow states, '[d]istances within lived-space depend strongly on how a man feels at the moment ... lived-space depends on a man's present disposition' (Bollnow 1961: 38). For example, the walk to fetch water may seem shorter than the return journey carrying a heavy weight. Second, conceptualising space as absolute effectively removes the human being from consideration. Abstract, mathematical conceptualisations of space do not prefer any one point in space to any other. This, Bollnow argues (1961: 32), is not the case with human, lived spaces, which always take their 'distinct coordinating zero point [from] the place of the living man in space'. Each person is the centre of her or his own universe.

Discussions of time inevitably require discussion of space, since the two are inextricably linked. While space is discussed in more depth in Chapter 4, a practice theory understanding of the relationship between space and time is introduced here.

What is space-time?

The relationship between space and time exists not only in objective space-time, in that everything must happen somewhere and some when, but also in human activity and practices; therefore, it is not possible to separate time and space when discussing the social world. The Kantian, dualist distinction between time and space, which left space on the lesser side of the time/space dichotomy, led to space being undervalued by scholars outside of the field of geography (Merriman, 2012). However, any conceptualisation of time as absolute inherently prevents its association with space, which is necessary for understanding the social world. Practice theorists link time and space into unified time-space, or space-time, by arguing that all interactions in time and space involve human beings (May and Thrift 2001).

Since space-time emerges from human interactions, it needs to be considered in terms of subjective experience. While objective space and time can be linked into dynamic, objective space-time, as in Einstein's theory of relativity (Hawking 1988: 33), understanding time and space in their subjectivity is equally and perhaps even more important for understanding the human world (Schatzki 2009), particularly so when the social world is conceptualised as located in practices (Schatzki 2002).

In order to distinguish between objective and subjective space-time, the terms space and time can be replaced by spatiality and temporality. Experiential **spatiality** is defined as:

> the world around (an actor) in its pertinence to and involvement in human activity. This world is pertinent to and involved in human activity in providing a platform for, and comprising entities that have places in, human activities.
>
> (Schatzki 2009: 36)

Experiential **temporality** is tied to human understandings of past, present and future. Whereas, objectively, the only time that can be said to exist is the present, human action is both future-oriented and affected by experience of the past. Seeing time dimensionally, as temporality, fixes an actor at the nexus of an affecting past and a potential future, allowing for deeper understanding of human actions in the present (Schatzki 2009).

Spatiality and temporality are mutually constitutive; inextricably linked by future-oriented human activity that affects how human beings organise the world spatially.

Space and time must, therefore, be considered together as a unified concept. Whether rendered 'with the obfuscatory hyphen in "time-space", the opaque ampersand in "space and time", the total collapse of "timespace"' (Merriman 2012: 14) or, as here, space-time, time and space are given meaning by understandings of the lived experience of the people in the times and spaces concerned. As Shove and colleagues state:

> ... spatial and temporal coordinates do not merely define the settings and scenes in which practices are enacted. Arrangements of time and place are structured by past practices and are themselves relevant in structuring future pathways of development and/or diffusion. In this role, they act like elements [of practices] in that they constitute media of aggregation and storage, holding the traces of past practice in place in ways that are relevant for the future, and for the perpetuation of unequal patterns of access.
>
> (Shove, Pantzar and Watson 2012: 134)

This section has argued that consideration of time and space is important for understanding the social world. Time and space are shown to be both objective and subjective, giving rise to a multiplicity of conceptualisations. The relationship between objective and subjective time and space is mutually affecting; consideration of the one without reference to the other is limiting or even, perhaps, impossible. Seeing time and space subjectively, in the form of temporality and spatiality, is necessary for understanding human activity. From this conceptualisation stems the possibility of looking at how different space-times change in relation to the practices and activities that generate them.

The next section considers occupational therapy as a social practice, looking at how it has evolved into its present form through an iterative process of performances over time; each of which entails goals, tasks, projects, purposes, emotions and normative assessments of what constitutes a correct or successful occupational therapy practice performance. All past performances of occupational therapy have left a legacy by structuring subsequent practice performances and affecting understandings of what occupational therapy (as a practice) is and could be.

The role of the occupational therapist

This section discusses time in relation to how occupational therapy roles are structured, how time is used and who makes decisions about the occupational therapist's time use.

Teleoaffectivities

Practice performance is always shaped by some kind of intent. Each time a person acts, it is with an end in mind and motivated by particular values, moods and feelings (Schatzki 1996). Every practice entity, such as occupational therapy, includes purposes and affective dimensions that motivate and shape performances. For example, one of the stated purposes of occupational therapy is 'to enable people to participate in the activities of everyday life' (WFOT 2012); and one of the affective values of occupational therapy is that everyone has a right 'to engage in a range of ... activities to enable them to maintain health, to flourish and create' (Trimboli 2017: 466). The word

teleoaffectivity was coined by Schatzki (1996) to refer to the totality of teleological (goal-directed) and affective (value-related) orders associated with a practice. Teleoaffective structures are the 'hierarchized orders of ends, purposes, projects, actions, beliefs, and emotions' that link the doings and sayings of an integrative practice (Schatzki 1996: 100).

Teleoaffectivity introduces a time dimension into practice. According to Schatzki (2006), a practice includes in itself the past, present and future; and all three are simultaneously present in practice performance. We always do things with a particular future in mind, even if it is only the enjoyment of a cup of tea and a temporary escape from the project one should be working on. Performing a practice takes us towards the future by changing things about ourselves and our space, however tiny those changes. Practice performances not only create the future but also, necessarily, contain the past. The practice comes from somewhere in space-time: we learned it at some point, watched others doing it, planned it and repeatedly performed it ourselves until it became a habit.

The day-to-day practices of occupational therapy

The profession of occupational therapy is maintained by the practice performances of occupational therapists, in their different jobs all over the world. What all of them are doing emerges from the past, is performed in the present and contributes to shaping the future. This conceptualisation of occupational therapy as a practice in time aligns with the occupational therapy theory of 'becoming through doing and being' (Wilcock 2006: 147); what we do now shapes what we become.

The practice of occupational therapy includes a wide variety of activities, which may or may not look like therapy. For example, when the occupational therapist asks a client to make a cup of tea, it can be for the purposes of assessment but can also be a means of providing a holding space-time, during which a purposeful but informal conversation can take place. The casual onlooker may not see that the primary purpose of the activity is to work towards reaching therapeutic goals rather than to produce a cup of tea (Creek 1996).

What the occupational therapist does in any particular instance is shaped by many factors: clients, setting, available resources and other people's expectations, including the non-therapy requirements of managers. Objective time is finite; requirements to take on generic or administrative tasks necessarily reduce the time available for doing occupational therapy. What occupational therapists do every day, therefore, as part of their work, is shaped by the particular demands made on them by the organisations and structures within which they are employed.

Given that each performance of occupational therapy is shaped by time and context, what the practitioner does on a day-to-day basis tends to be based on pragmatism rather than ideology. The occupational therapist does mainly what is required by employers, clients and significant others within the structures of the work setting, as discussed in Chapter 2. Occupational therapy intervention may be subject to constraints, set by the service, on time, space and scope; for example, home visits or follow-up sessions are often not mandated in the acute hospital setting. In statutory services, it is rare for practitioners to have full professional autonomy to choose their work focus and practices; however, most seek a reasonable compromise between their professional values and goals and those of employers and funders. This may be harder at some times than at others, depending on the extent to which the goals and values of the employing organisation are congruent with those of the occupational therapist. Being conscious of the organisational goals, values and motivations their work is expected to serve allows occupational therapists to seek opportunities for better alignment (see Box 3.1) in order to serve the best interests of patients or clients.

Box 3.1   Aligning the values and goals of occupational therapy with the employing organisation

An occupational therapist employed in an acute hospital works within a medical frame of reference and is expected to conform to the requirements for rapid intervention and discharge. The goals of occupational therapy must be phrased in terms that the organisation and colleagues recognise and value: this may result in a more reductionist, impairment-focused approach than the profession professes.

The duration of therapy in the acute setting is likely to be determined by the logic of medical treatment and pressure for discharge, unless a case can be made for longer interventions. For example, a person admitted to the hospital after a stroke will often be discharged when medically stable, allowing no time for them and their relatives to learn how to manage residual problems.

Where medical and managerial cultures are dominant, making the case for a longer hospital stay requires the therapist to demonstrate how their work links with concepts and goals prioritised by the organisation, such as improving clinical outcomes and reducing the likelihood of readmission. In the case of the post-stroke patient, the occupational therapist could frame intervention in terms of reducing the future risk of pressure sores or aspiration pneumonia. Data meeting the evidence standards of medical managers (e.g., findings from clinical research) and administrators (e.g., cost-effectiveness studies) will greatly strengthen the therapist's case.

The challenge for occupational therapists in such situations is to remain true to their professional identity and goals, while also applying such positioning strategies. Ultimately, one would hope to influence healthcare institutions towards a more multidisciplinary vision of health, but existing power bases and entrenched medical culture may make this a long-term prospect.

It is the small, daily practice performances of occupational therapists around the world that take the profession forwards into the future. If these day-to-day practices are determined, to a large degree, by the social, political and economic structures within which occupational therapists work, then the future of the profession may not remain congruent with its own values and ideals. The challenge for practitioners is to stay centred in professional values and vision, while translating these for a different paradigm. This struggle plays out through the dimension of time in the occupational therapist's everyday work.

Time spending and managing

As described above, time can be seen in many different ways, both objective and subjective. Subjective, or lived, time is about experiencing a practice through unfolding processes, sequence, associated values and the evocation of changing feelings; as when the practitioner is working face-to-face with a client. Objective time is the flow and pace of events that can be measured by the ticking of a clock: it is what we are thinking of when we speak of spending or managing our time, a finite resource with boundaries external to the practice or the performer.

Since objective time is finite and a scarce resource, the occupational therapist must make choices about how it can be managed and rationed. However, as explained in the last section, the therapist may have limited autonomy to choose how time is used. For example, there may be demands from funders and employers to account for time spent, meet performance targets and demonstrate that daily practice is directly serving the goals of the organisation (see Chapter 2 for further discussion of performance targets).

What occupational therapists do every day is necessarily shaped by influences other than the teleoaffectivities of the profession itself. Most occupational therapists are paid for the time they spend working rather than for deliverables or outcomes, meaning that time equates to money in a direct way. What is done in paid-for time can be determined largely by the purchaser's goals and intentions. Being paid, and hence being able to continue practising as an occupational therapist, is dependent on aligning with the goals and values of someone with funds.

The financial arrangements for healthcare vary across the world, and health economics research has demonstrated how different payment mechanisms shape the practices of providers and professionals (McKenna et al. 2017), as illustrated in Box 3.2.

Box 3.2   How healthcare funding influences time use

In a private sector, fee-for-service setting, time use is determined by what can be billed for. This, in turn, is specified by insurance companies or similar. Occupational therapists working in an insurance-funded healthcare system can only provide the specified interventions. Those in private practice must organise their work in a way that brings in the fees they need to survive. It is inevitable that certain services will be privileged or disincentivised by the funding structure. For example, multidisciplinary discussions and teamwork are difficult to fund on a fee-for-service basis, which therefore tends to promote fragmentation and professional competition for available funds rather than collaboration, sometimes to the detriment of the patient.

Occupational therapists working in the public sector, funded by governments, receive a salary regardless of the amount of time spent seeing patients. However, high caseloads may constrain the time that can be spent with each patient. Where a given population is entitled to receive certain state-provided services, the management of time is aimed at fulfilling these entitlements, on behalf of the government.

Different imperatives and constraints are in place where occupational therapy services are funded by non-governmental agencies or donors. While such funding may provide opportunities for occupational therapists to pursue their professional goals beyond what is possible in government or private sectors, it comes with its own constraints. Availability of funds is dependent on alignment between donor priorities and occupational therapy capacities and goals. Funding tends to be short-term (projects of one to three years), often with heavy demands for monitoring, evaluation and reporting. Time spent on governance activities can cut heavily into the time available for doing occupational therapy. Donors may be hesitant to fund salaries at full cost, so that an occupational therapist's time can be spent juggling multiple projects and funder requirements, in between looking for the next source of income.

Being a profession

The issues discussed so far, of autonomy and teleoaffectivity, speak to what it means to be a profession and raise the question of whether or not occupational therapy can be considered a profession. Occupational therapy emerged as a profession at the beginning of the 20th century, a time when unmarried, educated women were looking for useful work outside the home (see Chapter 1). The term **profession** is used to refer to a particular type of social practice that is defined by certain features (Hugman 1991; Clouston and Whitcombe 2008), as shown in Box 3.3.

Box 3.3   Features of a profession

Representative professional body, for example, college, council, association, federation
Specialised knowledge and skills
Salaried
Control over education
Power to determine professional roles and responsibilities
Autonomy to make clinical decisions
Responsibility for professional standards
Professional identity and social status
Job and/or career security

These criteria indicate that professional status is a variable social position that depends significantly on social, economic and political contexts and on the existence of structures that support professional practice, including funding.

It might be argued that, because occupational therapy evidences only some of these features, it has not achieved full professional status. There are several reasons for this, including changes in social, political and economic structures, power relations with other professions (Clouston and Whitcombe 2008) and the structure of organisations within which occupational therapists practise (Schatzki 2002). This means that occupational therapy might be viewed as a profession in some countries and not in others, at some times but not at others or only in particular places.

Further, as described in Chapter 2, the rise of managerialism on a global scale has eroded some aspects of the professional status of many professions, including occupational therapy, leading to reduced autonomy; less security (e.g., job, salary, pension rights, sick leave); less control over education, and being subsumed into the category of allied health profession, for the purposes of state recognition and registration, rather than being a separate entity (Clouston and Whitcombe 2008).

Social understandings of occupational therapy have not necessarily kept pace with how the profession has changed. In the minds of many people, including other healthcare professionals, occupational therapy is still associated with a particular time and mode of working: that is, with the early 20th century use of crafts as therapeutic media. In situations where the profession has never been associated with crafts, such as social services, primary care or community development, it is seen to be concerned with the ordinary and everyday and, therefore, based on common sense rather than specialised knowledge (Clouston and Whitcombe 2008).

The first section of this chapter looked at the big picture of occupational therapy practice over time: where the profession came from and where it might be going. It claimed that occupational therapy exists in the practices occupational therapists perform every day, all over the world, and considered what (and whose) teleoaffectivities might be guiding these practices. The governance of the profession's practices and goals was examined from the perspective of how time is spent, managed and accounted for.

This section focused on the role of time in structuring occupational therapy practice: what occupational therapists do in time, who determines time use and how that impacts on practice. Occupational therapists might argue that their teleoaffectivities are more aligned with the focus of this section than the first one, but we are frequently caught between two sets of goals and values. In such positions, we need to rethink our professional purpose and what we are doing in practice.

The final section of this chapter explores the everyday work of occupational therapists and aspects of professional reasoning around temporal dimensions of practice.

Time in occupational therapy practice

As described above, objective time, the finite number of minutes, hours and days available for practice performances, is often governed in work settings by management requirements, such as number of patients to be seen, hours to be billed for and non-therapy activities to be completed. All of these activities compete for time with the occupational therapist's profession-specific practices. In Chapter 2, it was shown how time use is a common focus for managerial intervention and control.

While such parameters might be outside the control of the individual practitioner, it is still necessary to think about how to work most effectively within them. Given limited therapy time and a large catchment population with diverse needs, how do occupational therapists prioritise and ration what we do? The kinds of decision that have to be taken include who we see first, what activities we focus on, how we make these decisions and, importantly, what effect these decisions may have on the people who use our services.

This section considers the multiple layers of time-focused reasoning needed in occupational therapy practice. Throughout the section, a case study of services for children with cerebral palsy in rural South Africa is used for illustration. Cerebral palsy (CP) is a leading cause of childhood disability and can involve multiple impairments, including difficulties with movement, cognition, hearing, vision and communication. Children and adults with CP may have complex and long-term healthcare needs, including rehabilitation and assistive devices. This case study describes services provided for this group by a rehabilitation team based at a government-run district hospital in a rural area of KwaZulu-Natal province, South Africa. The case is developed in four parts, each one illustrating different aspects of time-related reasoning in occupational therapy practice.

Case study 1.1: Making decisions about time use

The multidisciplinary rehabilitation team, which includes occupational therapists, provides both hospital-based and community services, covering the full age range from neonates to the elderly, and the full spectrum of physical and mental health conditions. Their catchment population is 120,000 people, living in one of the most deprived districts in the country. The team currently has on their books around 160 clients living with CP. The time available for one-on-one intervention is extremely limited, so decisions have to be made about how best to balance the needs of this group (people with CP) against other demands on the team. At present, children with CP are largely seen on monthly outreach days at primary care clinics, which are more accessible to many families than the district hospital. In this context, appointment systems do not work well, and clients simply turn up when they can. Depending on how many clients arrive on a given day, the therapist may have less than half an hour to spend with each child.

Conventional treatment for this client group includes neurodevelopmental therapy (NDT), which is taught at a basic level in South African occupational therapy undergraduate education programmes. During outreach clinics, many therapists attempt at least a short period of hands-on treatment for each child because 'this is what occupational therapists do'. However, evidence suggests that such treatment, even when delivered by skilled and experienced practitioners, requires high intensity (dosage and frequency) in order to be effective. In studies that show positive effects for therapy based on motor learning principles, therapy is provided at least once a week (often more), over several months (Novak et al. 2020). On the current service platform, such levels of input are not possible and the occupational therapist's approach must be reconsidered.

A logical shift is from direct treatment to skills transfer: adopting the role of a **trainer/educator** and teaching caregivers to carry out simple therapeutic activities themselves. Group interventions, with the therapist acting as a **facilitator**, may build on caregivers' own strengths and develop a support system between families facing similar challenges. Taking this a step further, selected caregivers may be trained as parent facilitators, who can provide more skilled and active support to other families, based on their own experience. The occupational therapist may then take on the roles of **supervisor** and **resource person**, supporting the parent facilitators' work. At the community level, an **advocate** role may be needed to address gaps in support services and facilitate access to resources, for example, by approaching local taxi drivers and owners to negotiate acceptance of children with disabilities as passengers.

Role reasoning

The concept of role reasoning was developed by Sherry and Oosthuizen (2017) for a course at the Department of Ergotherapie, at the University of Antananarivo in Madagascar. Occupational therapists may take on a variety of roles, depending on setting, strategy and need. While therapist (or clinician) is the most obvious role, others include manager, trainer/educator, facilitator, consultant or advocate, as described above. Role reasoning is a process of clarifying goals and responsibilities, setting boundaries, negotiating relationships and activities with others, and thinking strategically and ethically about what we do (and don't do).

Considerations of time are vital in identifying the best role to adopt in particular circumstances. A therapist on a fixed-term contract or voluntary placement must consider what is possible in the time available, based on an understanding of the temporal characteristics of the processes involved. This may include, for example, the time required to enter a new community, build trusting relationships and understand a different culture.

When the occupational therapist has the autonomy to determine which roles to take, the following questions can inform the choice of role in particular situations:

1   **Referral:** Why am I here? Who has asked me? What do they see as the problem?
2   **Situational analysis:** From an occupational therapy perspective, what are the problems/issues to be addressed?
3   **Who am I responsible to?** Who do I represent? What other roles do I hold?
4   **What is my mandate/scope?** Which issues are within and which are outside it?
5   **What resources are available?** (Including my time and funding)
6   **What skills and knowledge do I have in this area?** Should others be involved along with/instead of me?

Different roles require different levels of engagement over time. For example, a therapist may engage with clients in a relatively short-term intervention, such as acute rehabilitation after hand surgery, or over a much longer time period (continuous or intermittent), such as working with adults with degenerative neurological conditions. The intensity of involvement may also vary over time with the same client: for example, during acute rehabilitation post-head injury, a client may be seen daily (or more) in an inpatient rehabilitation unit. After discharge home, the client may be followed up weekly, monthly or less frequently in their home or as an outpatient. In contrast, a manager's role is generally continuous and consistent over time, providing day-to-day service oversight and looking after such functions as human resources, monitoring, evaluation and financial management. A consultant may enter a service, community or programme for a specific project for a much shorter time period (a few months or even weeks, for example, when conducting a programme evaluation) and once this task is complete her role is at an end.

Case study 1.2: Considering the temporal realities of service users

The above section considered therapist time in the design of effective and equitable services. This is not enough in itself: services impose time demands on clients and their families that must also be considered by service providers.

Women in rural southern African communities typically carry the bulk of the household workload, from growing food and carrying water and fuel, to caring for children and the elderly. Where infrastructure and services are lacking, these tasks can be both physically demanding and time-intensive, resulting in experiences of time poverty (Arora 2015). These are not only practical realities but are also embedded in cultural values and expectations: a 'good' woman is one who works hard for her family. In Zulu culture, women and girls must be up before sunrise to begin their tasks, showing that they are not lazy, and should be home before sunset; while men and boys may get up later and stay out after dark without disapproval.

Meeting social expectations may be especially important at certain times or stages of life. A newly married woman (or *makhoti*) traditionally lives with her husband's family for the first few years of marriage and must work particularly hard to gain the approval and acceptance of her in-laws.

Caring for a child with a disability can be extremely time-consuming. Everyday tasks of feeding, dressing and bathing tend to take longer, so that additional time for carrying out an occupational therapy home programme may not be available. Where the mother is also a *makhoti*, she may not have control over how her time is spent. Where family attitudes to a child with a disability are negative, it may be beyond the mother's power to do more than the essentials for her child. Taking the child for therapy may also have significant time implications for the household since travel and waiting times can render this a whole-day exercise.

Without insight into these realities, therapists might see caregivers as non-compliant or uncaring when therapy instructions are not followed or appointments kept, and these judgments can result in the breakdown of the relationship between caregiver and service. An understanding of both lived and objective time in the lives of children with CP and their families is therefore essential to providing acceptable and effective services.

Occupational therapy practice and lived time

Consideration of lived time moves beyond the notion that practices simply vie for a share of finite temporal resources, to reveal how 'time is something that practices "make"' (Shove, Pantzar and Watson 2012: 129). For example, the practice of baking bread produces a temporal sequence that includes a time to turn on the oven, a time to mix the ingredients, a time to let the dough rise and a time to put the bread in the oven and take it out. In this way, practices create time by giving rise to timings and sequences that are necessary for the successful performance of the practice, even though these timings may vary during different performances.

Therapists work with many human processes that have or create their own time in this way. Physiological processes, such as wound healing, may have fairly defined time features which must be thoroughly understood in planning and carrying out rehabilitation: for example, the healing of a repaired flexor tendon in the hand dictates a strict protocol of splinting and controlled mobilisation through the stages of recovery. Processes of human development unfold in known sequences, and this knowledge is applied in work with children and infants with neurological, physical or environmental challenges. A growing scientific understanding of the 'first 1000 days' (UNICEF 2017) is focusing therapists' work in Early Childhood Intervention (ECI). Less defined and predictable is the unfolding of psychological, emotional and social processes: the stages of grieving after a diagnosis of disability; the process of a therapeutic group and the progression of community entry into a new setting. An understanding of these unfolding processes, their sequence, determining factors and possible trajectories is central to professional reasoning across the scope of occupational therapy, from the treatment of a single individual to the development of the profession in a country or region.

Case study 1.3: Life stage considerations

By definition, the neurological damage underlying CP occurs at some time between conception and the second birthday. This period is increasingly understood as critical in all aspects of human development; neurological damage at this early stage will disrupt and permanently alter the trajectory of physical, cognitive, sensory-perceptual and socio-emotional development. Accepted treatment approaches used by occupational therapists for cerebral palsy, such as NDT, depend on a detailed understanding of normal developmental sequences and the ways in which these may be altered by CP in its different forms. Both the sequencing and the timing of developmental milestones inform clinical reasoning in the treatment of individual children with CP.

The timing of therapy within the child's lifespan is a further consideration. It has been shown that children with CP achieve 90% of their gross motor potential by age 5, with the greatest development during their first two years (Rosenbaum et al. 2002). At a programme level, efforts are therefore needed to identify children with neurological problems as early as possible, and there is evidence-based justification for prioritising early intervention in the allocation of scarce rehabilitation time and resources (McIntyre et al. 2011).

Unfortunately, in the rural context described above, children begin compulsory schooling in the year they turn seven, and not all will attend preschool before this. Children with barriers to learning may therefore only be identified and referred for treatment after the critical period for early intervention has passed. Another cause of delayed referral is the common practice of first seeking either traditional or faith-based healing for a child born with a disability. Taking the child for medical treatment may be seen as demonstrating a lack of faith, either in God or the ancestors, therefore this only happens when other methods have failed. The emotional process of coming to terms with the child's condition can only begin once the hope of a miraculous cure is given up, often delaying the caregiver's readiness to engage with therapy. Insight into these processes is crucial for therapists in shaping how they approach and build relationships with families.

Past, present and future

Objective time is unidirectional; it flows forwards from past to future (Adam 1990). This unidirectional flow means that human beings tend to perceive time as having three dimensions: past, present and future. In objective time, these dimensions are discrete and contain events that either once existed (past), currently exist (present) or are yet to exist (future). This is important when trying to understand the unfolding of historical events, such as the brief history of occupational therapy given in Chapter 1, or when considering the implications of the flow of such events for possible futures, as discussed in Chapter 9.

When considering human experiences of time and activity, it is useful to think of past, present and future as '*features* of activity' (Schatzki 2009: 37, original emphasis). From this perspective, 'the three dimensions of activity appear together so long as a person acts. If activity ceases, the three disappear together' (Schatzki 2009: 37). This understanding of time in human activity is teleological; that is to say, human activity is directed towards particular ends (Schatzki 2010). In the moment of doing (the present), people are applying knowledge and experiences of the past, in search of desired, future outcomes.

The flow of time has implications for the ways in which occupations are performed, by groups and by individuals. What people expect and value in the performance of everyday occupations is powerfully shaped by 'how it's always done' or 'how I did it before my injury/illness/and so on'. Carrying out the most mundane occupations in a familiar and customary way connects the person in the present to all others who are doing it the same way and to all who have gone before and done it the same. Ways of doing things become traditional, linking past, present and future in the performance.

Different cultures vary in their relations to past, present and future and in how these are perceived. Hofstede, Hofstede and Minkov (2010) proposed a set of six continua that can be used to describe and compare different cultures, one of these continua being relative emphasis on past, present and future. Modern Western cultures tend to be future-oriented, with a focus on progress; they embrace change and innovation and emphasise working towards goals and desired futures. Cultures indigenous to Africa and other regions may be more past-oriented, with a strong value given to tradition and long-standing ways of doing things. Belief systems around ancestors, as a continuous presence and active force in daily life, may be powerfully linked with a past-focused worldview. Customary practices are a means of anchoring oneself within a group and a history, maintaining connection to others, both living and deceased, and building continuity from the past to the present and future.

Occupational therapy was originally developed within a Western worldview, so that working towards a possible future, or avoiding an unwanted one, is inherent in the therapeutic process. The teleoaffective structures of occupational therapy practices are intentionally organised with this future orientation, and the skill of identifying manageable goals and organising therapy around these is central to what is considered high-quality occupational therapy. The range of possible futures associated with the clinical prognosis of a given condition informs where goals could be sited, as do available opportunities in the therapeutic context.

Case study 1.4: Orienting therapy towards the future: Goals and decisions

Focusing rehabilitation on defined goals is recognised as crucial to effective therapy with children with CP (Novak et al. 2020). Client-centred practice requires that such goals are set collaboratively and aligned to the client's own values and priorities. When mothers of children with CP are asked their goals, the most common replies involve their child being able to walk, talk and attend school. For children with moderate to severe CP (Gross Motor Function Classification System Levels IV and V), these goals may be unrealistic, especially in the context described in this case study, so parental expectations need to be sensitively navigated. Helping the mother come to terms with this reality, while sustaining her hope, motivation and engagement, is a challenging process. Parent facilitators, who can speak from their own experience and demonstrate an intelligible future for such families, may be better placed than therapists for this role (Saloojee and Bezuidenhout 2020).

What happens in therapy needs to be clearly related to what is valued by the family. Change in children with CP tends to be slow, and continued investment in re-habilitation depends on caregivers being able to connect every contact session with their own goals and priorities. For example, explaining how sitting prepares the body for standing and walking can help motivate a mother to work on this with her child at home. Connecting independence in toileting with being able to go to school may encourage her to let her child try to pull up his pants himself, even though it takes longer.

This process of orienting practices within occupational therapy towards a hoped-for future is not always straightforward. Setting and working towards personal goals is culturally familiar and valued in Western societies, especially among those in higher socio-economic brackets. In Western cultures, future orientation, individualism and a sense of control over one's own future are key underpinnings to the concept of goal-setting. Cultures strongly oriented to the past may find goal-setting less natural, while religious and cultural beliefs about the role of God, the ancestors or other spiritual forces in determining events can produce a fatalistic rather than self-determined view of the future. People living in poverty, with high levels of daily uncertainty, low levels of control over their circumstances and immediate survival concerns, may be necessarily focused on the present and short-term future rather than on a more distant future (Box 3.4). Such life experiences may also produce low levels of self-efficacy.

Box 3.4   Family decision-making: Immediate needs versus future orientation

An elderly woman was admitted to a rural hospital in South Africa, with a suspected spinal fracture. The X-ray machine was broken, making it impossible to know whether or not the fracture was unstable, and there were no corsets or spinal braces available. While staff waited for the machine to be fixed, the lady was placed on strict bed-rest.

The day came round for monthly pension payments, which required recipients to go in person to the pay point for thumbprint ID. This woman received an old-age pension, which was the main income for her family. The occupational therapist arrived in the ward to find five or six men and women standing around the woman's bed, waiting for her to come with them to the pay point.

Together with the doctor, the therapist explained to the family that there was a risk of spinal cord injury and paralysis if the woman was moved. The healthcare workers urged them to let her remain in bed but could not enforce this. The family needed the pension to be able to eat that day so, in spite of the risk of causing lifelong disability, they took their injured relative to fetch the money.

Such situations can be hugely challenging for occupational therapists and other professionals because the decisions made by service users and their families seem to violate our core values: disability prevention, individual autonomy and even human rights. It would be tempting to intervene more forcefully to protect the patient, or at least to judge harshly the family making the decision. But such responses would disregard the different realities in which they live: not only the exigencies (and subsequent time orientation) of extreme poverty but also the collective culture in which the family and its relationships are placed above the needs of the individual. In that situation, the occupational therapist also had to think ahead to the consequences of conflict with the family: relational breakdown could block the patient's future access to services, as well as potentially placing blame on this woman for any negative consequences for her family of not accessing the pension on that day.

This example illustrates how time orientation is bound up in the lifeworlds of service users and how this can play out in occupational therapy practice. Time is shown to be closely bound up with cultural (and professional) values, creating an imperative for therapists to interrogate their own assumptions and try to understand those of their clients/ patients.

Summary and conclusion

This chapter explored how practice theory conceptualisations of time may be applied to occupational therapy, both as a profession (globally and locally) and in the design and conduct of day-to-day therapy services. Considering time (particularly as space-time) brings up a range of issues tied to the themes of this book: the professional standing of occupational therapy, the ways in which the day-to-day practices of occupational therapists are shaped and how these practices, in turn, shape the profession as a whole, both now and into the future. We have also attempted to illustrate some of the many temporal dimensions of practice, as subjects for professional reasoning in context. The next chapter takes up the space dimension of space-time to extend these ideas further.

References

Adam, B. (1990) *Time and social theory*. Cambridge: Polity.

Arora, D. (2015) Gender differences in time-poverty in rural Mozambique. *Review of Social Economy*, 73(2): 196–221.

Benner, A.D., Wang, Y., Shen, Y., Boyle, A.E., Polk, R., and Cheng, Y.P. (2018). Racial/ethnic discrimination and well-being during adolescence: a meta-analytic review. *American Psychologist*, 73(7): 855–883. 10.1037/amp0000204

Bollnow, O.T. (1961) Lived space. *Philosophy Today*, 5(1): 31–39.

Clouston, T.J., and Whitcombe, S.W. (2008) The professionalisation of occupational therapy: a continuing challenge. *British Journal of Occupational Therapy*, 71(8): 314–320.

Creek, J. (1996) Making a cup of tea as an honours degree subject. *British Journal of Occupational Therapy*, 59(3): 128–130.

Encyclopedia Britannica. https://www.britannica.com/science/spectroscopy/Radio-frequency-spectroscopy#ref620572. Retrieved 12 July 2021.

George, J., Morton Ninomiya, M., Graham, K., Bernards, S., and Wells, S. (2019) The rationale for developing a programme of services by and for indigenous men in a first nations community. *AlterNative: An International Journal of Indigenous Peoples*, 15(2): 158–167.

Hawking, S.W. (1988) *A brief history of time: from the big bang to black holes*. London: Bantam Press.

Hofstede, G., Hofstede, G.J., and Minkov, M. (2010) *Cultures and organizations: software of the mind*, 3rd ed. New York: McGraw Hill.

Hugman, R. (1991) *Power in caring professions*. Basingstoke: MacMillan.

Loy, D.R. (2001) Saving time: a Buddhist perspective on the end. In: J. May and N. Thrift (eds.) *Timespace: geographies of temporality*. London: Routledge. 262–280.

McIntyre, S., Morgan, C., Walker, K., and Novak, I. (2011) Cerebral palsy – don't delay. *Developmental Disabilities Research Reviews*, 17(2): 114–129.

McKenna, H., Dunn, P., Northern, E., and Buckley, T. (2017) *How health care is funded*. London: The King's Fund. Online at https://www.kingsfund.org.uk/publications/how-health-care-is-funded. Accessed December 2021.

Massey, D. (1999) Space-time, "Science" and the relationship between physical geography and human geography. *Transactions of the Institute of British Geographers*, 24(3): 261–276.

May, J., and Thrift, N. (eds.) (2001) *Timespace: geographies of temporality*. London: Routledge. 10.4324/9780203360675

Merriman, P. (2012) Human geography without time-space. *Transactions of the Institute of British Geographers*, 37(1): 13–27.

Novak, I., Morgan, C., Fahey, M., et al. (2020) State of the evidence traffic lights 2019: systematic review of interventions for preventing and treating children with cerebral palsy. *Current Neurology and Neuroscience Reports*, 20(3). 10.1007/s11910-020-1022-z

Purcell-Khodr, G.C., Lee, K.S., Conigrave, J.H., Webster, E., and Conigrave, K.M. (2020) What can primary care services do to help first nations people with unhealthy alcohol use? A systematic review: Australia, New Zealand, USA and Canada. *Addiction Science and Clinical Practice*, 15(1): 1–21.

Rosenbaum, P., Walter, D., Hanna, S., et al. (2002) Prognosis for gross motor function in cerebral palsy: creation of motor development curves. *Journal of the American Medical Association*, 288(11): 1357–1363.

Saloojee, G., and Bezuidenhout, M. (2020) Community-based peer supporters for people with disabilities: lessons from two programmes. In: H. Kathard, A. Padarath, R. Galvaan and T. Lorenzo (eds.) *South African health review 2020*. Durban: Health Systems Trust. 89–97.

Schatzki, T.R. (1996) *Social practices: a Wittgensteinian approach to human activity and the social*. Cambridge: Cambridge University Press.

Schatzki, T.R. (2009) Timespace and the organisation of human life. In: E. Shove, F. Trentmann and R. Wilk (eds.) *Time, consumption and everyday life*. Oxford: Berg. 36–48.

Schatzki, T.R. (2002) *The site of the social: a philosophical account of the constitution of social life and change*. University Park: Pennsylvania State University Press.

Schatzki, T.R. (2005) The sites of organisation. *Organization Studies*, 26(3): 465–484.

Schatzki, T.R. (2006) The time of activity. *Continental Philosophy Review*, 39(2): 155–182.

Schatzki, T.R. (2010) *The timespace of human activity: on performance, society, and history as indeterminate teleological events*. Plymouth: Lexington Books.

Sherry, K., Dabula, X., Reid, S., and Duncan E.M. (2020) Decolonising qualitative research with rural people with disabilities: lessons from a cross-cultural health systems study. *International Journal of Qualitative Methods*, 19: 1–11.

Sherry, K., and Oosthuizen, A. (2017) Role reasoning in occupational therapy. Unpublished course notes, Department of Occupational Therapy, Faculty of Medicine, University of Antananarivo, Madagascar.

Shove, E. (2009) Everyday practice and the production and consumption of time. In: E. Shove, F. Trentmann and R. Wilk (eds.) *Time, consumption and everyday life*. Oxford: Berg. 17–34.

Shove, E., Pantzar, M. and Watson, M. (2012) *The dynamics of social practice: everyday life and how it changes*. Los Angeles: Sage.

Southerton, D., and Tomlinson M. (2005) '"Pressed for Time": the differential Impacts of a "time squeeze"'. *Sociological Review*, 53(2): 215–239.

Tan, J. (2021) Suicide prevention: a sociocultural approach to understanding suicide among inuit–issues and prevention strategies. In: R. Schiff and H. Moller (eds). *Health and health care in Northern Canada.* Toronto: University of Toronto Press. 255–273.

Trimboli, C. (2017) Occupational justice for asylum seeker and refugee children: issues, effects, and action. In: D. Sakellariou and N. Pollard (eds.) *Occupational therapies without borders: integrating justice with practice*, 2nd ed. Edinburgh: Elsevier. 460–467.

Tuan, Y.F. (1977) *Space and place: the perspective of experience.* London: University of Minnesota Press.

UNICEF South Africa (2017). The first 1000 days: the critical window to ensure children survive and thrive. Pretoria: UNICEF. Online at https://www.unicef.org/southafrica/media/551/file/ZAF-First-1000-days-brief-2017.pdf. Accessed January 2022.

WFOT (2012) *Statement on occupational therapy.* Online at file:///C:/Users/User/AppData/Local/Temp/Definitions-of-Occupational-Therapy-from-Member-Organisations-LINKS-Update-11022020.pdf. Accessed May 2022.

Wilcock, A.A. (2006) *An occupational perspective of health*, 2nd ed. Thorofare, NJ: Slack.

Yalmambirra (2000) Black time ... white time: My time ... your time. *Journal of Occupational Science*, 7(3): 133–137.

4 Space-time, place and working contexts

Kate Sherry and Anri-Louise Oosthuizen

Introduction

The concept of space-time was introduced in Chapter 3, with a focus on occupational therapy unfolding through time as a profession and practice. This chapter looks more closely at the spatial aspects of space-time.

Occupational therapy persists as a practice entity across space and time, with its own locations, histories and trajectories. Some of the history of occupational therapy is presented in Chapter 1, which describes the development of the profession in Europe and North America, and in Chapter 8, which includes the history of occupational therapy in Brazil. The performance of occupational therapy also takes place in space and time; that is, each performance is located in a particular place, occurs at a particular time and has a specific duration. For example, an occupational therapist leads an activity group (practice performance) in the day room of a secure unit (location) every Wednesday afternoon from 2 pm (time) until 4 pm (duration).

The places where occupational therapy is practised form nexuses of related practices (Blue and Spurling 2017). For example, an occupational therapist working in a hospital is part of a nexus of connected practices that includes the doings and sayings of patients, relatives, nurses, doctors, managers, porters, other occupational therapists, cleaners, administrators, physiotherapists, radiographers and many others. In another place, such as a refugee settlement, the contribution of the occupational therapist is part of a nexus of the practices of displaced persons, local and international aid workers, local communities and so on. In any place where occupational therapists work, they find themselves connecting, co-operating, competing, collaborating, communicating and co-ordinating with many other groups and practices.

The multiple practices that constitute a place for action, such as a hospital, have to negotiate how the available space and time are allocated; including which practices are given priority when time is limited and how space is organised to accommodate different practices. For example, the occupational therapist leading the Wednesday activity group on a secure unit has to finish the group on time because the day room is needed for afternoon tea. The many practices of the hospital, therefore, are connected and interdependent in space and time. Some of the dimensions of this interdependence are explored in other chapters; such as *power* in Chapter 2, *marginalisation* in Chapter 6 and *resources* in Chapter 7.

This chapter begins by explaining some key concepts from practice theory concerning space, illustrated with a case study of an everyday public space where different practices occur. Objective and lived space, spatiality and place are explored, as well as

DOI: 10.4324/9781003016755-4

macro-level factors influencing practice spaces. Existing ways of thinking about space in the occupational therapy and occupational science literature are briefly reviewed, with reference to what practice theory might add. The next part of the chapter explores the spaces where occupational therapists work and what this means for their practice(s). The final section considers how occupational therapists might use practices intentionally to shape new spaces for their work. Case studies are drawn from a variety of settings to illustrate these ideas.

What is space?

It is impossible to separate human experiences of time from human experiences of space because future-oriented human action structures how human beings organise the world spatially. For example, the physical design of hospital buildings evolves to accommodate new healthcare needs and practices. Nonetheless, Chapter 3 presented a justification for exploring time and space as distinct phenomena.

In Chapter 3, we saw that there are many ways of thinking about time. Equally, there are different ways to understand the phenomenon of space. **Objective or mathematical space** can be seen as a three-dimensional container, bounded by height, width and depth, in which no point is uniquely privileged over any other. For example, each of the six sides of a cube is the same size and all are equidistant from the centre; there is no difference between them. In **lived space**, the relative position of things is determined by the perspective of the observer, in the same way that someone standing in the doorway of a room will see the layout and contents of the room differently from someone standing in the middle. Lived space is not merely physical: it includes social, emotional, cultural, personal and other dimensions.

The term **spatiality** refers to the experiential quality of space. It is 'the world around (an actor) in its [relevance] to and involvement in human activity' (Schatzki 2009: 36): spatiality is space as it is seen from the point-of-view of people doing things. Spatiality also has a temporal dimension, since prior uses of space inform what people do with and in that space in the present and the future, and provide a base on which human activities take place (Schatzki 2009: 36). The activities in which people engage provide the motivation for structuring the world spatially in the ways they do: 'In the end, teleology [purposeful action] underlies spatiality because spatiality is the pertinence that objects around have for human activity, and the pertinence of the world around for activity ultimately rests on the matters for the sake of which people act' (Schatzki 2009: 38). In other words, human beings understand spaces as spaces in which to do x, y and z, and this requires a conception of what is to be achieved in a particular space, be it treating a patient or drinking a cup of coffee. It follows that the way we perceive and interpret the world around us is based on what is important to us, and on what we need and want to do in it. The example given in Box 4.1 illustrates these ideas.

As Schatzki (2009) suggested, for each person in this example, different features of the space are pertinent. The young labourer is focused on the distance between this piece of pavement and his place of work; the people around him are obstacles to be negotiated as fast as possible. The two nannies are most concerned with their conversation and, in a secondary way, with negotiating the physical space on the pavement to push two prams side-by-side, sometimes giving way to other pedestrians. The space is familiar to them and they hardly notice it. The young woman divides her attention between her phone and her anticipation of coffee with her friend; half-alert to the people around her and the safety of her handbag. To the homeless man, the pavement is living space and the low wall, unnoticed by others, is his favourite seat. For the jogger, the pavement is part of her running route and its slight downhill slope means she often clocks her fastest kilometre split here, if it is not too crowded. The emotional and mental states of these actors are completely different, as are their preoccupations, goals and concerns (their teleoaffectivities). Some feel a sense of belonging and ease in this space, others do not.

The pavement example illustrates a practice theory understanding of space as **relational** (Hui and Walker 2018). The space described is experienced and used by each actor in relation to their past experience, current activities and concerns, personal characteristics and many other dynamics. It also exists in relationship to other spaces, as disparate as an upmarket coffee shop, a playground, a crowded shack, a building site and a war-torn foreign country. Most significantly, the space is defined in relation to the practices taking place within it. Through the way the various actors use the pavement, it has become a place for sitting, socialising, getting to work or exercising.

As the example in Box 4.1 illustrates, a space can be the setting for the performance of multiple practices. As another example, a grassy outdoor space can be a racecourse, arable land, a building site, a football field, a meadow or the site of a music festival. However, different features of a space constrain the practices that can be performed there and influence how they are performed. For example, football played in an indoor gymnasium has different rules, kit and organisation from football played on a large, grassy field.

Box 4.1 A pavement as both objective and lived space

On a stretch of pavement in a suburb, a number of people are walking. All occupy the same physical location, at the same time, and all are moving from one place to another.

A young woman in a stylish summer dress is strolling along, checking her mobile phone. She has just parked her car and is on her way to meet a friend at the trendy coffee shop around the corner. A young man, perhaps the same age, is striding with purpose in the same direction. His clothes show him to be a labourer and he carries a backpack. He has come from the station, having caught an early train from the township on the outskirts of the city where he lives. The walk from the station to his place of work is almost three kilometres and, because of train delays, he is late. He is a casual day-labourer and, knowing that being late could cost him his job, he walks fast. As he passes the young woman, she glances up quickly. The city has a high crime rate and she is habitually aware of the people around her.

Two women, slightly older, pass the young man, going in the opposite direction. They move slowly, chatting as they push prams containing two small children. Like the labourer, they got up early to catch public transport. They are nannies for two of the wealthy families who live in this suburb and are on their way to the park, where they will meet other nannies they know. They will sit on the grass and pass the time together while the children play. Back at their own homes, their own children must stay inside when they are not at school because gang violence makes the streets unsafe.

An elderly man with tangled hair shambles along muttering quietly to himself. He is homeless and is going nowhere in particular. He sits down on a low wall in the sun to smoke a cigarette and asks another man passing for a light. This man stops and chats for a few minutes. He is an official at the magistrate's court down the road and often sees the old man around the area. As he lights a cigarette of his own, he recognises another man passing on the pavement as an asylum-seeker, whose case was heard in the court the day before and who is now faced with deportation. The man is on his mobile, speaking in French with a desperate tone to his voice. A middle-aged woman in Lycra jogs past them, headphones on.

All these people occupy the same objective space: a short stretch of pavement, beside a moderately busy street, in a well-to-do suburb. For all of them, it is a sunny Tuesday, around 8: 30 in the morning. They are all apparently doing the same physical activity: walking from one place to another. Yet the lived spaces they occupy in that moment are entirely different. Some are at work, or on their way there, while some are at leisure. In occupational therapy terms, for each person, the action of moving along that pavement forms part of a completely different occupation.

Lived spaces are not only located in the physical world but can be, for example, social, cultural, political, virtual, discursive or conceptual. The young woman checking Facebook on her phone is operating in a virtual social space. The asylum-seeker's situation is determined by national and international factors in a political space. The nannies' companionship takes place within a particular socio-cultural space. Ideas are developed, shared, and contested in discursive spaces. Knowledge is organised and categorised in conceptual spaces. All these types of space can be places for social practices.

Space and place

A space becomes a **place** when people ascribe to it particular meanings and value (Tuan 1977). This meaning and value come from their experiences of being in that place and from the activities performed there (Pink 2012). This means that a place acquires its placeness for people because of the practices associated with that place: ' … space is itself defined by what goes on within it' (Shove, Pantzar and Watson 2012: 132).

The arrangements and meanings of a place, in turn, affect what happens in it, to the extent that it is associated with a particular practice or practices. What occurs now in a given space is dependent upon what happened there previously, and what will occur there in the future depends upon the practices being performed there now. On our piece of pavement, the court official joins the homeless man for a smoke-break, other commuters follow the route from the station and the nannies meet their friends going to the park. The nature of space is therefore contingent and dynamic, as practices emerge, continue, change or die away. Perhaps the nannies and prams discourage the runner, who changes her route to allow a faster pace or the cloud of cigarette smoke deflects non-smoking commuters to the opposite pavement.

In occupational therapy practice, there was a time when hospitals were places for treatment and houses were places for living everyday life. At some point, occupational therapists began visiting people at home, so their houses became places for assessment and intervention. Once a house was experienced as a place where occupational therapy could be performed, this became a present reality and future possibility. In places where occupational therapy is new, its practices may seem odd and out of place. In a healthcare facility where no rehabilitation has previously been provided, a therapist who gets people with strokes out of bed is chastised for 'disturbing the sick people'. With time (and hopefully some successful treatment outcomes), the ward becomes a place for rehabilitation as well as for nursing; and rehabilitation practices become part of the place.

Places constantly change as elements come together in different ways in the performance of different practices. A grassy field may be a place for grazing cattle for 11 months of the year and the site of a music festival for one month. Similarly, occupational therapists also conceptualise occupations and places as mutually shaping: the way an occupation is performed is influenced by the place where it is performed and, conversely, each occupational performance changes the place. As practices evolve over time, the elements that make up the practice change (see Chapter 8) and this impacts the place of performance. For example, a modern music festival on a greenfield site requires more and different provisioning from a 1960s music festival (Allen 2018).

While lived space and place are formed, as it were, from the inside out (by the practices that take place within them), both spaces and practices are also shaped by the broader contexts within which they exist. In the following section, the situated nature of practice spaces is further explored.

Nexuses of practice

In examining the spaces in which practices are performed, it is vital to understand the broader context and nexus of practices from which they emerge. As mundane as our pavement scene may appear, the actors' experiences of this space are shaped by broader social, political, historical and economic forces. The city is Cape Town, South Africa, a region still heavily marked by the racialised spatial policies of the Apartheid regime. This suburb was once designated a *white* residential area and, less than 40 years ago, people of colour could only enter such areas if they were employed there and carried certain paperwork (the so-called *dompas*). Residents of this suburb are still overwhelmingly white and middle- or upper-class, while people of colour in Cape Town, both locals and immigrants from other African countries, still largely occupy outlying townships and informal settlements.

These outlying spaces house a continual influx of poor people from elsewhere in the country and the continent, drawn by the better services and (comparatively) greater opportunities for employment in this city. Unemployment is extremely high and casual labourers, such as our young man, are endlessly replaceable; hence his anxiety about being late for work. Those who manage to get jobs travel long distances daily, on unreliable public transport. The young woman's alertness to potential mugging is not unfounded but the relative safety of this setting contrasts with the gangland home of the nannies, which in turn seems safe to refugees from civil wars in countries to the north. The contrasts of one of the most unequal countries in the world are starkly visible here. The practices available to the different actors in this pavement space are shaped by a complex political, historical and socio-economic context.

People partition spaces into places in many ways, including national boundaries, administrative jurisdictions, sacred sites, private property and common land. Often, it is the most powerful group that determines the meaning of a space and who are allowed access to it, as in the Apartheid-era land distribution laws, mentioned above. The exercise of power to control who has access to a space and how it is used constitutes space as a commodity. Throughout human history, people have colonised spaces, exploited them for profit, been driven out of them, confined to them and barred from entering them.

The Canadian sociologist, Titchkosky (2008: 41), wrote of 'discourses of competition for scarce resources, hetero-normative expectations, colonizing powers, and neoliberal demands' that control who has access to certain spaces and places. (The issue of access is explored in more depth in Chapter 6.) Indigenous people groups, who held different conceptualisations of land that did not include ownership, particularly hunter-gatherer cultures, such as the Khoisan in South Africa and the Aborigines of Australia, were rapidly overcome by the colonisers who displaced them (Van Wyk 2016). The high political sensitivity of land restitution processes in post-colonial states reflects the multi-dimensional significance of place. The issues at stake are not simply economic ones: land is invested with cultural, spiritual, historical and socio-emotional value as well; and the same space may hold layers of significance and meaning for different groups, giving rise to competing claims.

Space, place and occupational therapy

Different ways of thinking about space have arisen in occupational therapy and occupational science over time. In this section, we briefly outline some key strands of thought to date, before turning to explore what a practice theory understanding of space might add to the field.

Space in occupational therapy and occupational science literature

Occupational therapists use words such as *setting*, *environment* and *context* when referring to the places where people perform their occupations. These are all described as *places for action* (Creek 2010), a conceptualisation not dissimilar from the practice theory idea that places are constituted by practices (Shove, Pantzar and Watson 2012). The significance of space (in which people perform occupations) is well established in occupational therapy theory and practice, although concepts have evolved and been contested over time.

In its simplest form, space is seen by occupational therapists as the environment or context in which an occupation is performed. The influential *Person-Environment-Occupation* (PEO) model proposes that appropriate fit between the three named elements is what enables occupational performance (Law et al 1996). The interventions of the occupational therapist may target any of the three elements to enhance that fit; for example, developing the skills of the person, adapting the occupation or modifying the environment. The *International Classification of Functioning, Health and Disability* (ICF) (WHO 2001), widely adopted by occupational therapists around the world, analyses the environment (physical, social, political, cultural, virtual, etc.) in terms of barriers and facilitators to participation by the individual. Both these theoretical frameworks assume a clear separation between the person and the space they occupy, tending to see space as a container for what the individual does and minimising the interrelations between the two.

This tendency to separate person and space has been critiqued in a body of work applying transactional perspectives, largely based on the ideas of the American philosopher and educationalist, John Dewey, to the study of occupations (see, e.g., Cutchin and Dickie 2013). These authors take issue with the individualism assumed in theoretical frameworks such as those cited above, arguing that people and their environments are not so easily separated: they interpenetrate, co-define and co-constitute each other (Cutchin, Dickie and Humphry 2006). From this perspective, occupation-as-entity and occupation-as-performance encompass the complex transactions of person and context, in which each is both active and acted upon, and both change as a result.

Transactional perspectives lend themselves particularly to the study of social spaces, in which people are most clearly at one with their environment through their relations with other people. Dewey's focus was a humanist one, centred on people's capacity for thought, action and choice as they engage with situations, solve problems and ultimately work towards a better society. He noted that people's choices are shaped both by circumstances and by perceptions of the possibilities available to them but paid little attention to how these circumstances and perceptions come about (Rudman and Huot 2013). Critical scholars within the transactional turn in occupational science have drawn on other theorists, such as Bourdieu and Foucault, to deepen understandings of how historical, social, political and economic forces shape the situations in which people find themselves, and the courses of action they perceive to be available to them (e.g., Rudman and Huot 2013; Galvaan 2015). More recently, Deweyan occupational scientists have also expanded their focus on the social, shifting to a greater community orientation in line with Dewey's ideas on development and social change (Cutchin, Dickie and Humphry 2017). At the same time, the body of work identifying as *transactional* within occupational science has adopted an increasing array of theoretical perspectives and interpreted the challenge of transcending individualism in a widening variety of ways (Josephsson 2017).

Precise comparisons of transactional occupational science and practice theory are difficult, given that both are diverse groupings of related work rather than unified theories in themselves. They share certain starting points, specifically with respect to how space is conceptualised relative to actor and action. Both challenge the false dichotomy of person and environment and draw attention to the complex interrelating of the two through action. Both consider how space (especially social space) shapes the range of actions open to an individual, according to their relations with that space, and their resulting sense of what can and should be done within it [reflecting practice theory's roots in cultural theories, also favoured by transactional scholars (Reckwitz 2002; Nicolini 2012)]. However, transactional occupational science still tends to begin with people, whether as individuals or as communities, and considers the situation (environment or space) in terms of what it means for them: the focus is on the relationship between person/people and space.

By contrast, practice theory begins with occupation-as-practice, framing people and space as elements of practices. A practice theory understanding of space centres on a dynamic relationship between space and occupation, the implications of which are worked out in the rest of this chapter. Practices are seen as the site of the social, rather than human minds, interactions or communication (Reckwitz 2002). A practice theory understanding of occupation is not structured around human lives and social processes but follows the lives of practices (as entities and performances) over time and space. In this way, practice theory perhaps goes further than transactional occupational science in transcending the individual.

The topic of space within the study of occupation is a complex one, with much recent interest and a burgeoning literature. This section has provided only a short overview of key issues, with reference to the possible contributions of practice theory to this study. The remainder of the chapter explores some practical workings-out of a practice theory understanding of space in the work of occupational therapists.

Space and occupational therapy practice

Applying practice theory conceptualisations of space to the work of occupational therapists sheds light on how practices evolve in different settings and on what the things we do may mean in the particular setting (space-time) where we are. The following case study takes an apparently simple question, asked of an occupational therapist in a variety of spaces/places, revealing how a practice takes on different meanings, implications and forms, depending on how it is embedded in context.

Case study 1: 'Do you do massage?'

Boxes 4.2–4.5 describe the different ways in which one occupational therapist responds to the question 'Do you do massage?', depending on the spatial-temporal context of the interaction.

Box 4.2   'Do you do massage?' Context 1

I am at a social occasion and someone asks what I do. The familiar blank look at the words 'occupational therapist' is followed by the question: **'Do you do massage?'** leading almost inevitably to the half-joking 'My neck is a bit sore, can you … ?' I am mildly irritated by the repetitiveness of this encounter, the minimisation of what I do and the tired joke (which sometimes borders on a pick-up line). My response is a polite laugh, a blunt negative and a rapid transition to another topic.

Box 4.3   'Do you do massage?' Context 2

I meet a new patient or colleague in a South African clinic setting, who is trying to understand the difference between occupational therapy and physiotherapy. They ask, **'Do you do massage?'**. Here, explaining the technical role distinctions is important, not least because interprofessional politics over scope of practice make the question a sensitive one. Technically, as an occupational therapist, I might use scar massage, manual oedema mobilisation, neurodevelopmental preparation techniques and other modalities that resemble massage but, officially, in this setting, 'massage' is the remit of physiotherapists. I say so.

Box 4.4 'Do you do massage?' Context 3

I am the new (and first) occupational therapist for a small island community, doing my best to explain my role and what I can offer. People on the island have had exposure to physiotherapy, social work and psychiatry but occupational therapy is new. They ask, **'Do you do massage?'**. From habit, I begin by saying 'no': I am not there to run a massage service, which could easily swallow much of my limited time. But soon I realise this response might be a mistake. People are slow to trust outsiders and reluctant to visit the clinic with personal matters. Coming with a stiff neck, however, is perfectly acceptable. While we apparently deal with the tight muscles (obviously staying well within my clinical capabilities), there is a chance to chat, to build a relationship and so get on to the underlying problems. I change my answer and begin to tell people that 'yes, I do massage'.

Box 4.5 'Do you do massage?' Context 4

I am an external consultant on a project to develop community-based services for children living with severe neurological disability, in East and Central Africa. During my time with a group of physiotherapists and physiotherapy assistants in Cameroon, they ask me, 'When you work with these children in your country, **do you do massage?**'. They want an outsider's opinion on the effectiveness of this kind of treatment. I know that some training for community workers in South Africa teaches simple muscle preparation techniques under the name of 'massage', so I answer accordingly. But it soon emerges that, in Cameroon, massage is associated with 'therapists' of variable training (there is no registration system for allied health professionals in the country), who practise an extremely forceful, painful form of manipulation on children with cerebral palsy (CP). They charge high fees, which dedicated parents pay, although the screams of their children often drive them out of the house during the therapist's visits. This group of physiotherapy staff has worked hard to educate parents about the ineffectiveness and possible danger of this treatment. I quickly revise my answer to their question, in strong support of their anti-massage efforts.

In each of these four examples, 'massage' has different connotations and constitutes a slightly different practice, with different implications for the role of the occupational therapist. The same question requires a different answer in each situation, based on a careful reading of the practice in context. This example illustrates how practices within occupational therapy may change their meanings and implications when transferred into different settings, and points to the dangers of uncritically replicating ways of doing occupational therapy from one place to another.

Unlike many (if not most) professions, occupational therapy is not characterised by a universal, recognisable set of activities or procedures, nor is it tied to a specific, characteristic space or setting. Being concerned with the everyday lives of clients, doing occupational therapy may look like nothing more than making a cup of tea or playing with a child. There are few special technologies or products to signal special knowledge, such as pills, X-rays or electrotherapy machines, and the spaces in which occupational therapy takes place may not be marked out from the home, community and workspaces of everyday life.

This lack of recognisable practices, spaces and materials to define the profession can be a significant challenge, both to outsiders (colleagues, clients, funders) and to occupational therapists themselves. Explaining what occupational therapists do is far from straightforward and the temptation to identify one's profession in terms of specific practices and settings is understandable. It is difficult to convey the logic that links activities as diverse as observing a child in a classroom, designing a bathroom adaptation for an elderly person, running a community awareness campaign and facilitating education planning in a refugee camp. What makes sense to do as an occupational therapist cannot be separated from the spaces in which one is doing.

Working in institutional settings

Chapter 2 described the alignment of occupational therapy with medicine during the 20th century, explaining the conceptual and pragmatic basis for this choice, as well as the tensions resulting from the alliance. Today, perhaps most occupational therapists across the world practise in medical settings, or at least within a biomedical frame of reference, and it might seem strange even to question such a positioning. In the previous chapter, Box 3.1 presented the example of an acute care setting and the ways in which an occupational therapist might need to frame their work within institutional structures: temporal, physical and conceptual. According to practice theory, spaces are shaped by the practices that take place within them and, in turn, shape what practices they can host in the future. This discursive relationship between space and practice is vividly experienced by occupational therapists working in healthcare institutions and other organisations.

To belong to a medical team means to adopt certain language, practices and behaviour. Wearing a uniform, working within a hierarchy, using acronyms, reading and writing in patient files, attending meetings and ward rounds and even participating in tea-room conversations are all practices that identify one as a team member. On the one hand, such performances act on relationships with colleagues and managers, recruiting professional recognition and inclusion. On the other hand, they present an image to service users that locates occupational therapy within the medical paradigm and triggers certain roles, expectations and behaviours within the therapeutic encounter. The patient is passive and compliant, the healthcare worker is an expert and success is measured in terms of the administration of a medication or procedure that effects cure.

This script may be at odds with the intentions of the client-centred therapist but can be difficult to reframe within a medical context. Most occupational therapists in medical settings have experienced the contradictions and disjunctures of working within such places. Unless or until occupational therapy has established its own space within the facility, where different expectations and practices operate, the fit is an uneasy one. Occupational therapy language is alien to the dominant discourse in the biomedical context, and values such as quality of life and meaningful occupation may be denigrated as 'nice-to-haves' but relatively unimportant beside the heroics of pre-venting death and curing disease. The dominant value systems translate into the or-ganisation of space and the allocation of resources within institutions, including remuneration and professional status. Consequently, there is a danger not only that occupational therapy services are side-lined but also that occupational therapists themselves lose focus and identity, as their practices conform increasingly to the medical paradigm.

Occupational therapists working in other types of institutions, such as law firms or schools, may have similar experiences in situating their work within the various spaces and everyday life of the setting. Practices must be intelligible to others within the institution; this will be shaped by what has been done there before and what else is being done in that space at present. Nonetheless, at the same time, therapists can carve out new spaces and places for themselves through the practices they undertake, as illustrated in Case study 2.

Case study 2: The battle of the chair

In a small rural hospital, rehabilitation services are being established for the first time. Occupational therapy is unfamiliar to most staff and almost all patients. People who are admitted after a stroke are kept in hospital while they are medically stabilised and are then sent home, often to remain in bed for the rest of their lives, waited on by family members. To both nurses and patients, the wards are spaces to be sick and being a patient means resting in bed.

The newly appointed occupational therapist arrives in the ward one day with the physiotherapist (also new) and they begin working with the stroke patients. At first, they simply help the patients to sit up and then to transfer into a chair beside the bed. The hospital is short of furniture but the therapists have found a perfect therapy chair in a storeroom: sturdy and upright, with arms and firm cushioning. One by one, the patients have a turn sitting out in the chair; but not without resistance from some of them, as well as from their family members. 'They are sick! Why are they being made to get up?' The nurses are equally displeased. 'Who are these new people [the thera-pists] and why are they disturbing the patients?'

The therapists persevere with their routine of getting each person up but, when their backs are turned, the nurses put the patients back into bed. The therapy chair dis-appears from the ward and turns up at the nurses' station, being used by a staff member. Patiently, the therapists retrieve the chair (there are others for the nurses to sit on, but these have wheels and will not work for rehabilitation) and try again.

This situation can be seen as a dispute over the space of the hospital ward: what it is for, and what practices are intelligible and acceptable there and by whom. The chair is a significant object within that space. To the therapists, it is a piece of equipment for rehabilitation. To the nurses, it is a place to rest and to fill out paperwork.

Gradually, there is a shift in the dynamics of the situation. The therapists build relationships with the ward staff and everyone becomes used to seeing 'sick' people getting out of bed without ill effects. The big breakthroughs come when patients learn to walk and to do things for themselves again. Families and staff see people they considered permanently paralysed regaining function. Not only have the practices that were considered acceptable within the ward changed but also the practices considered available to someone with a stroke are vastly expanded. By the following year, rehabilitation is an everyday part of the hospital space.

A practice theory understanding of space is invaluable for occupational therapists moving into new spaces and responding to changing societal needs and opportunities. Understanding how spaces emerge from practices and vice versa gives us a powerful lens for understanding what we do, and hope to do, in context. What works in one space might not make sense in another and the unthinking transplantation of practices may be at best ineffective or, at worst, damaging to the communities they aim to serve (Thibeault 2013). For example, the extended case study of CP services in Chapter 3 showed how attempts to reproduce conventional therapy (as taught at university and practised in urban and first-world settings) were rendered nonsensical by the temporal dimensions of the practice context. Although such inadequate interventions might be considered 'better than nothing' by providers, in reality, the costs to families of accessing those services might outweigh any possible benefit to the child with CP.

Reconsidering practice spaces

The work of occupational therapists may not always be best served by the typical spaces in which they practise, particularly when those spaces are linked to institutional settings, such as hospitals or clinics.

Moving our work onto new ground may offer completely new possibilities for action and impact. The following section again takes up the example of the rural CP service described in Chapter 3, this time focusing on the space aspect of space-time.

Case study 3: Space-time of the CP outreach clinic

This case study is in two parts, each describing how certain occupational therapy practices unfolded in the light of the spaces within which they were performed.

Part 1: The clinic setting

In the rural district described in Chapter 3, therapy services for children and adults with CP have chiefly been accessed at primary care clinics, where the rehabilitation team conduct outreach once or twice a month (per clinic). Distances are large in this area and the clinics are much nearer to where people live than the district hospital, although for many the travel time and cost may still be considerable. Since rural life and transport are not predictable enough to make appointment systems practicable, outreach days are run on a first-come-first-served basis. This means caregivers must often leave home very early in the morning (having first attended to the water, fuel and food needs of the household for the day) and may wait several hours at the clinic before being seen. Part, if not all, of the journey to the clinic will be on foot and, since the terrain is too rough to make wheelchairs feasible as transport, clients with more severe CP must be carried. (It is for this reason that attendance at the clinic often decreases after a child is five or six years of age when she becomes too heavy to make the journey). Thus, by the time clients and their caregivers arrive at the clinic, they have been up since very early in the morning and have often had an arduous journey. Transportable food may be a challenge, so both caregivers and children are tired and hungry.

Meanwhile, the therapy staff begin their day at the hospital with early morning team meetings, rapid handovers of ward patients and the often-challenging process of securing transport, which, even when booked well in advance, is often changed or cancelled at the last minute. The hospital vehicles are poorly maintained and not all have the 4 × 4 capabilities required by the local terrain. Breakdowns, flat tires and getting stuck in thick sand are common events, making the journey out to the more distant clinics, which can be up to two hours' drive, especially interesting.

When therapy begins at the clinic, both staff and patients have already covered significant ground, physically and emotionally, to be there. The clinic space itself is usually cramped and two or three staff may need to treat patients in the same room. Waiting areas are often overcrowded so that patients spill out into the clinic grounds, not always with protection from the weather, which may bring anything from burning sun to heavy rain. The hours available for service provision are constrained by travel time on either side, often leaving therapists with no more than 20 minutes per patient.

Thus is the space-time in which occupational therapy is provided for children and adults with CP shaped: not only is the physical space confined but other factors, including the geography and infrastructure that determine the journey to reach it and the total time available, result in a treatment setting characterised by disruption, distraction and exhaustion for all parties. In this context, high-quality engagement between therapist and client is virtually impossible; and it is uncertain how such an encounter can yield any benefit worth the family's investment of time and effort in getting there.

Part 2: Alternative spaces

After several years, the rehabilitation team working in this district recognised the limitations of the outreach clinic setting and began experimenting with alternatives. When regular outpatient services shut down, in 2020, in response to the COVID-19 pandemic, staff began visiting children and adults with CP in their homes. It quickly became clear that taking the encounter into a different space dramatically changed what could be done. Although, in some cases, the therapy team still needed to travel considerable distances, their clients did not. Not only did this save them a great deal of time and money but they entered the engagement in a far less stressed and exhausted state. A relaxed, comfortable child presents completely differently from a hungry, irritated one, allowing the therapist to gain a more accurate picture of his functioning and to engage with him more meaningfully.

Seeing the child in her home also gave the team insight into her everyday life context and that of her family, surfacing many relevant, practical issues that were invisible in the clinic. The physical space available at home might make sense of why an assistive device was never used (too cramped or inaccessible entranceway), while furniture (or lack thereof) might explain feeding methods and positioning of the child during the day. Visible markers of poverty, the presence of other household members with specific needs (e.g., elderly parents, also in need of care) and sources of water and fuel (hence household labour demands) further explain where caregivers are *coming from* in their attitudes and actions towards the child. Seeing the household in context, therapists realised the need to act according to family priorities, not their own. This could mean assisting with access to social welfare, connecting other family members with needed healthcare or advocating with tribal leaders, in order to deal with concerns that currently supersede the needs of the disabled child. Once the necessary preconditions were in place (e.g., food security), families were far more likely to engage with rehabilitation.

Instead of a single caregiver, the whole family, often plus curious neighbours, could be present at the session. Interventions could therefore include discussion and education with the child's larger support system. In multi-generational households, the caregiver who brings a child to the clinic might not be a decision-maker in the household; conversations with elders and heads of families made it possible to address attitudinal barriers and mobilise influence in the child's favour.

Not least important was the shift in roles and interactions afforded by the home space. Outside the physical bounds of the health system, family members were far less constrained by patient–doctor scripts and they could take a more active and confident role in therapeutic interventions happening on their own ground. Further, the relational value of healthcare workers making the effort to visit people in their own homes helped build trust and openness. Once therapists began adapting their expectations and priorities according to the real-life context of the family, their effectiveness increased dramatically, as did the satisfaction of families with services and that of therapists in their own work.

Taking CP services into people's homes proved to mean far more than simply shifting the delivery point of a given intervention. It fundamentally changed the practices that make up those services and hence what could be achieved with children and their families. The commonly used term 'service delivery' in itself assumes that healthcare and rehabilitation are like packages: predetermined, neatly wrapped and independent of their environment, needing only to be handed over to those in need. This metaphor denies the complexity of effective occupational therapy interventions, often to the detriment of context-appropriate service planning and management. A practice theory understanding of space makes this clear.

Shaping spaces to enable practices

So far, this chapter has demonstrated how practices take on different meanings in relation to the spaces in which they occur; and how the spaces in which occupational therapy happens can constrain or support its quality and goals. The skill of reading practices in relation to space is fundamental to professional reasoning. We have argued that spaces emerge from the practices taking place within them and, in turn, become places where those practices can happen in future. In this final section, we explore how spaces may be intentionally configured and developed by therapists to foster the practices we wish to see.

Case study 4: Practices and pedagogy: Training for contextually appropriate occupational therapy in Madagascar

The University of Antananarivo began its occupational therapy education programme in 2015, with the explicit goal of producing graduates able to develop and provide contextually appropriate and culturally relevant occupational therapy services for Madagascar. This meant not only training students in internationally accepted theory and practice but also equipping them to weigh and interpret this in the light of their own society and national context. Authentic practice is impossible without acknowledging when theory and tools are created in different spaces from the indigenous space. An evaluation measure, for example, is created with a specific population in mind. It is created in a specific country, where there are particular resources, activities, value and modes of reasoning: standardisation is, at best, standardisation in context. Much time in the occupational therapy course is spent discussing where tools and methods were developed, how context and activities might be different there, whether these tools and methods are locally relevant and which parts of them apply. This critical reflection allows not only for situated practice but also for deep reasoning.

Developing such professional reasoning skills is fundamental to student training. Students entering the occupational therapy programme at the University of Antananarivo come from a wide variety of cultures, some of which place a strong value on family hierarchy, others on the guarding of corporate peace. Both principles can make critical and reflective questioning and commenting seem counter-intuitive. Hierarchical social structures are further reflected in the classroom, both at school and university: the teacher is the expert and the job of students is to absorb what they are taught and repeat it when asked. Students might ask questions to collect information (e.g., 'Can you explain?'), but will almost never ask 'why?'.

From a practice theory perspective, the classroom begins for the students as a place for listening, writing and repeating. The occupational therapy programme needs to create a different kind of learning space, in which new practices (questioning, reflection and reasoning) can take place. To do this, the new practices need to be introduced, practised and repeated until they become habits; and until their performance makes the classroom a place where these things can continue to be done. This process must be repeated for every new intake of occupational therapy students. With time, this has been refined into a distinct pedagogical approach.

As with every activity, graded opportunity optimises success. In a hierarchical and collectivist society, this means beginning with students working together before being expected to carry out practices individually. In the first semester of an occupational therapy course, students might be asked to form groups and ask their questions of one another before formulating questions to be asked of the lecturer (i.e., up the hierarchy). In this way, the practice of questioning is first done in a social group of peers, then as a group consensus expressed by a representative and, finally, with individuals asking freely for themselves. Setting up this sequence through all aspects of the course creates spaces that at once build the practice of asking questions and simultaneously acknowledge the culture that directs the skill.

The types of questions to be asked are also graded, starting with concrete or factual questions, such as *how* to do something, before moving on to more abstract ones, such as *why* something should be done. Social learning is vital and the lecturer must model the different practices before requiring students to try them out for themselves; at which point peer modelling and feedback can occur. For example, in order to teach self-questioning as a reflective tool, the lecturer speaks through her own self-questioning in different situations, in front of the class, before having them self-question.

Understanding learning practices in relation to space has also produced strategies for developing students' professional identity. Studying on a medical campus, where most professional courses favour the medical model, it is important for occupational therapy students to stake their claim to being occupation-based. For example, during the foundational activity analysis module, students are sent to brush their teeth in the school's washroom. As other students observe and ask what they are doing, they get to explain occupational therapy, with human activity as its centre. The use of public space during teaching thus allows consolidation of professional space within the medical school. At the same time, students are being prepared for working in healthcare institutions, where similar explanations and 'space-making' will be necessary.

The example given in this case study describes just one way in which an understanding of the mutually constituting nature of spaces and practices can inform effective occupational therapy work.

Summary and conclusion

This chapter has explored how the space aspects of space-time, as theorised in practice theory, may be interpreted by occupational therapists, especially those working in emergent or alternative contexts. A skilful reading of practices in relation to space has been highlighted as essential to strong professional reasoning. Even where occupational therapy has been long established in its role, there is a need to consider how institutional space and competing values and professional cultures may shape its daily practices. If occupational therapy as a profession consists in what therapists do every day, these daily practices are far from trivial. The spaces in which they unfold must be understood not only as their immediate setting but also as situated within broader historical, cultural, political and socio-economic contexts.

The next chapter considers where the profession of occupational therapy is located at the present time and the social issues that it could be addressing.

References

Allen, M.E.P. (2018) Understanding temporariness beyond the temporal: Greenfield and urban music festivals and their energy use implications. In: A. Hui, R. Day and G. Walker (eds.) *Demanding energy: space, time and change.* Cham, Switzerland: Palgrave Macmillan. 73–93.

Blue, S., and Spurling, N. (2017) Qualities of connective tissue in hospital life. In: A. Hui, T. Schatzki and E. Shove (eds.) *The nexus of practices: connections, constellations, practitioners.* London: Routledge. 24–37.

Creek, J. (2010) *The core concepts of occupational therapy: a dynamic framework for practice.* London: Jessica Kingsley.

Cutchin, M.P., and Dickie, V. (eds.) (2013) *Transactional perspectives on occupation.* Dordrecht: Springer.

Cutchin, M.P., Dickie, V.A., and Humphry, R. (2017) Foregrounding the transactional perspective's community orientation. *Journal of Occupational Science,* 24(4): 434–445.

Cutchin, M.P., Dickie, V.A., and Humphry, R. (2006) Occupation as transactional experience: a critique of individualism in occupational science. *Journal of Occupational Science,* 13(1): 83–93.

Galvaan, R. (2015) The contextually situated nature of occupational choice: marginalised young adolescents' experiences in South Africa. *Journal of Occupational Science,* 22(1): 39–53.

Hui, A., and Walker, G. (2018) Concepts and methodologies for a new relational geography of energy demand: social practices, doing-places and settings. *Energy Research and Social Science,* 36: 21–29.

Josephsson, S. (2017) A move for framing occupation as transcending the individual? *Journal of Occupational Science,* 24(4): 393–396.

Law, M., Cooper, B., Strong, S., Stewart, D., Rigby, P., and Letts, L. (1996) The person-environment-occupation model: a transactive approach to occupational performance. *Canadian Journal of Occupational Therapy*, 63(1): 9–23.

Nicolini, D. (2012) *Practice theory, work and organization: an introduction.* Oxford: Oxford University Press.

Pink, S. (2012) *Situating everyday life.* Los Angeles: Sage.

Reckwitz, A. (2002) Towards a theory of social practices: a development in cultural theorizing. *European Journal of Social Theory*, 5(2): 243–263.

Rudman, D., and Huot, S. (2013) Conceptual insights for expanding thinking regarding the situated nature of occupation. In: M.P. Cutchin and V.A. Dickie (eds.) *Transactional perspectives on occupation.* Dordrecht: Springer. 51–64.

Schatzki, T.R. (2009) Timespace and the organization of social life. In: E. Shove, F. Trentmann and R. Wilk (eds.) *Time, consumption and everyday life: practice, materiality and culture.* New York: Berg.

Shove, E., Pantzar, M., and Watson, M. (2012) *The dynamics of social practice: everyday life and how it changes.* Los Angeles: Sage.

Thibeault, R. (2013) Occupational justice's intents and impacts: from personal choices to community consequences. In: M.P. Cutchin and V.A. Dickie (eds.) *Transactional perspectives on occupation.* Dordrecht: Springer. 245–256.

Titchkosky, T. (2008) "To pee or not to pee?" ordinary talk about extraordinary exclusions in a university environment. *Canadian Journal of Sociology/Cahiers Canadiens de Sociologie*, 33(1): 37–60.

Tuan, Y. (1977) *Space and place: the perspective of experience.* Minneapolis: University of Minnesota.

Van Wyk, B. (2016) Indigenous rights, indigenous epistemologies, and language: (re) construction of modern Khoisan identities. *Knowledge Cultures*, 4(4): 33–45.

WHO (2001) *ICF: International classification of functioning, disability and health.* Geneva: World Health Organization.

5 The current position of occupational therapy theory and practice

Nick Pollard

Introduction

Over the last 100 years, the development of occupational therapy has been shaped by a variety of influences, as identified in Chapter 1. Much of the written history of the profession has considered its growth under the auspices of the medical profession but has not often considered other influences on its development. In many countries, the profession has been dominated by the sometimes patriarchal and controlling influence of medicine, which has determined the selection of entrants and educators, favouring middle-class women with practical skills. This has been particularly marked in the United Kingdom and its former colonies (Wilcock 2001; Joubert 2010; der Merwe and Rauch 2019; Orton 2021). Until the last few decades, the training of occupational therapists (many of whom are still in practice) was often conducted through systems administered through government health institutions. In the United Kingdom, occupational therapy schools developed within local voluntary hospitals, such as the Astley Ainsley in Edinburgh, and continued under the National Health Service from 1947. These arrangements offered national qualifications (Perryman-Fox and Cox 2020; Nancarrow and Borthwick 2021). More recently, and with a growth in demand for occupational therapists in many countries with expanding economies, the education of occupational therapists is moving to universities.

The profession has numbered strong and determined pioneers and champions amongst its members, such as Dr Elizabeth Casson, who trained as a medical doctor and advanced the profession in England; Eleanor Clarke Slagle, a social worker who established the profession in the United States, and Nise da Silveira, the Brazilian psychiatrist who set up the first occupational therapy programmes in Brazil (see, e.g., Wilcock 2001; Peters 2011; Peters, Martin and Mahoney 2015; Monzeli, Morrison and Lopes 2019). From the beginning of the profession, there has been a strong emphasis on the development and expansion of practice, whereas research and theoretical knowledge have tended to develop along narrower pathways.

In the United Kingdom, occupational therapy research often had to be self-funded or financed through social fund-raising events, while most of the early research into its benefits was carried out by doctors. In order to produce a research evidence base for practice, occupational therapists had to develop educational and supervisory structures, together with the means of dissemination that could support it. These structures were largely developed by the efforts of occupational therapists themselves, through their professional associations (Wilcock 2001). More recently, access to post-graduate programmes, research opportunities and the doctoral and post-doctoral agendas for

DOI: 10.4324/9781003016755-5

occupational therapists and other professions have tended to be ordered to the generic priorities of the health service employers who provide funding for students (Nicholls 2017; Pollard et al. 2020).

Chapter 2 set out the influence of managerialism on the profession in determining how occupational therapists can work within health and social care systems. As a consequence of these constraints, some of the fundamental questions raised about occupational therapy are not well explored: what constitutes meaningful and purposeful occupation; how does occupation relate to such social phenomena as class and culture, and why do occupational therapists tend to assume that engagement in occupation is positive, rather than acknowledging the full complexity suggested by psychological, anthropological and social science researchers? Some aspects of that complexity were discussed in Chapters 3 and 4, where we addressed occupational therapy as a social practice in time and space.

The limited scope of scholarship and research in occupational therapy perpetuates a narrow perspective of the current function and future potential of the profession. The hierarchical power structure of health services, and the bias of research agendas towards physical sciences, have left occupational therapy with a weak evidence base for the allocation of essential resources, such as premises or staffing. As a result, the times and spaces in which the social practice of occupational therapy may be found are easily overlooked and potentially misunderstood. Furthermore, occupational therapy, and the people that occupational therapists work with, may become invisible and unrecognised because the times and spaces where this work takes place are outside the purview of the dominant and self-perpetuating cultures of health and social care systems.

In Chapter 2, we explored how the interests of powerful groups, and the consequences of their dominance, prefigure the possibilities for action of those with less status and less power or capacity. An example is given in Box 5.1 of an occupational therapist advocating for her client's invisible occupational needs to be recognised by the funding authority.

Box 5.1 Occupational therapist as an advocate

An occupational therapist, based in the United Kingdom, worked with a client who had profound and multiple learning disabilities. The young man could only move his head and had to have extensive care and support to meet his basic needs; including PEG (percutaneous endoscopic gastrostomy) feeding, personal care, medication and physiotherapy.

The occupational therapist observed that the client did not have access to a satisfying range of activities; the only sensory activity to which he responded positively was having his hands placed in warm water. The therapist found a bathing cradle that could support him to take a bath, as he liked being submerged in water rather than just showering. However, before the bathing cradle could be installed, a ceiling track hoist had to be fitted in the bathroom.

Major housing adaptations are funded by the local authority so the occupational therapist applied to the Disabled Facilities Grant panel. The panel said that the adaptation was for therapeutic purposes and they could only provide funding for care.

In this situation, the occupational therapist could have said 'Well, the local authority says "no"' and left it at that. She may even have agreed with the panel that, in the context of scarce resources, the bathing adaptation was rather frivolous. Instead, the therapist chose to advocate for the client against structural barriers; to try to change the care system to fit the person, not the other way around. She took the position that access to meaningful activity comes under the Care Act, arguing her case with three different local authority managers.

After many months, funding was agreed and the young man will at last have access to an activity that he enjoys.

What this chapter is about

This chapter provides a bridge between the historical development of the profession described in the first part of this book and future developments laid out in the second part. It began with a summary of the factors identified in Chapters 2, 3 and 4 that shaped the development of the occupational therapy profession into a constellation of practice, throughout the 20th century. The next section explains what is meant by *a constellation of practice* and considers in more depth two of the global social phenomena that shaped occupational therapy: colonialism and social inequality. The third section discusses some of the major global social issues providing the context for the current and future practice of occupational therapy: climate change, inequity and health, sustainability and displacement. The final section explores where the profession of occupational therapy finds itself in the early 21st century, in terms of social and health needs, power structures, occupational therapy theory and emerging areas of practice.

Constellations of practice in the 21st century

Occupational therapy, or rather therapies, can be described as a community of practice. A community of practice is a term developed by Jean Lave and Etienne Wenger (1991) to describe processes of shared learning and knowledge exchange, either formal or informal, through which people can develop. Communities of practice can be associated with teaching and learning; for example, the acquisition of professional skills. Occupational therapists and other health professionals form communities of learning for continuing professional development activities, such as a journal club or lunchtime seminar; but other communities of practice are associated with community activities, such as a local history group or a Villages in Bloom society. A range of skills may be acquired through joining any form of organisation, as is clear throughout history; for example, in the way communities share knowledge and practices around food, hunting, cultivation and, ultimately, eating together (Jones 2007).

Communities of practice work through the ways in which people use their social identity to build social capital through the exchange of knowledge. People work together on real tasks, avoiding duplication through shared problem-solving and communication of ideas. The concept of communities of practice helps us to understand organisational behaviours and is particularly associated with the development of industries that require constant innovation.

Communities of practice can, in turn, be combined into constellations of practice (Wenger 1998), which are larger groupings of similar nodes of knowledge exchange. It is possible to recognise constellations of practice throughout human society (see example in Box 5.2). We can also see occupational therapy, or therapies, as a constellation of practice. For example, a national association of occupational therapists is formed of communities of practice that may be based around clinical specialisms, education or localities.

Box 5.2   A constellation of practice

A community writers' workshop can be seen as a community of practice in which members exchange their knowledge of writing techniques, literature and, perhaps, different methods of publishing. In turn, the writers' workshop may affiliate with a larger organisation, which combines with other workshops to more critically develop their writing through opportunities for publishing, meetings and events in a constellation of practice.

For example, many authors writing in the science fiction genre developed through communities of practice. One such group was called the *Futurians*, the most well-known of whom, Isaac Asimov (1980) and Knight (1977), authored or edited over 500 books and provided the base plot for popular films such as *I Robot*.

It is difficult to determine key influences on the development of a practice over the course of history, but the beginning points of a historical process always precede what we select as the starting point. We may choose to locate the starting point of occupational therapy at the founding meeting of the National Society for the Promotion of Occupational Therapy, in 1917, but the roots of the profession can be traced further back in time. Two areas of linked social practices that influenced the development of occupational therapy are briefly explored below and some of the social issues connected with them are identified.

The legacy of colonialism

The worldwide pattern of human development can be seen to have taken place to the benefit of some people while at enormous cost to others, through centuries of extraction of goods from colonised countries and necro-economic dominance (that is, an acceptance within the economic policy that many poor people will die earlier to provide wealth for a relative few) (Linebaugh and Rediker 2001; Montag 2005; McLynn 2011). This colonial development still shapes patterns of consumption in the 21st century, leading to a widening inequality gap between the richest and poorest people in the world (Oxfam 2022).

European colonialism tended to begin as private enterprise ventures, organised by companies seeking to exploit new territories. Traders sought to develop markets in commodities such as spices, slaves, gold, sugar, tea, coffee, cloth and minerals.

Governments followed in the wake of private investors: the British Empire, for example, became a means through which the powerful elites and middle classes in the United Kingdom could develop influence and gain wealth, while the working classes found work adding value to the raw materials imported from colonised countries (Black 2018). Traders in other developed nations vied for influence around the world; between them destabilising economies, destroying indigenous industries, exploiting local labour and transferring diseases and pests across continents, as they sought maximum profit (Linebaugh and Rediker 2001; Tharoor 2018).

The human damage, from both colonialism and resistance to it, is evident to this day. For example, Ireland's rate of migration has been far higher than other parts of the British Isles and its present-day population is far lower (Kenny 2017; Hickman and Ryan 2020). Political instability often persists in countries and areas that have endured colonisation, such as Haiti (Obregon 2018), Latin America and South-East Asia (Tharoor 2018; Shefner and Blad 2019). Much of the wealth extracted from colonised countries was spent by the elites who controlled it, but it also enabled 18th- and 19th-century European industrialisation (McLynn 2011; Tharoor 2018). This generated the wealth and tax revenues that funded public systems in the Global North, such as health services, state education and social welfare institutions.

The social structuring of inequality

Across the world today, governments aim to achieve economic growth that will sustain their popularity, while individuals want to amass personal fortunes by playing the markets with their existing resources (Varoufakis 2016; Andreff 2019). Greed, or self-interest to the exclusion of others, is a dominant feature of boom and bust capitalism in the 21st century. This was shown in the privatisation of public utilities in the United Kingdom; the selling of unsecured loans to home buyers with insecure incomes, and the growing power of oligarchs, who bought up public assets as they were sold off (Andreff 2019). Powerful banking corporations work to maintain the status quo by manipulating currency differences to stimulate demand for goods and shape the global economy. When interest rates are high, those people in poorer economies who are able to put their savings into property can borrow against their homes to buy goods that will sustain desired social practices; such as computers to support their children's education or better quality household goods. The money they owe can be sold on to other banks, in complex arrangements that mask the ultimate unsustainability of these loans (Varoufakis 2016).

The rhetoric of continuous economic growth, and the manipulation of facts to hide the reality of economic disparity, generate significant public distrust (Flinders 2021). Banks, corporations and international trade organisations can act as anti-democratic influences by working to promote a fluid market, with few policy controls, which they control to their advantage (Max-Neef 2010; Varoufakis 2016; Shefner and Blad 2019). The oligarchical and corporate powers involved become influential in governments around the world, that support these powers because they are too big to fail, even when many of them permit and facilitate criminal activity, such as money laundering on a huge scale (Andreff 2019).

The Chilean economist, Manfred Max-Neef (2010), argued that the global economy is set up to serve the short term, ultimately destructive interests of global trade organisations and very wealthy individuals, whose instituted practices seem to be outside effective regulation. The effects of this complex combination of powerful interests work against the possibility of sustainable development and risk exceeding the resources and capacity of the planet. Economic and political development are very different around the world but global connectivity produces a situation where dominant powers make macro decisions that affect everyone on the planet at the micro-level. Conversely, individual actions collectively impact the survival and the experiences of inequality and injustice of others.

Many governments and corporations acknowledge that the global economy and its relation to the environment have reached a crisis point, but, nonetheless, there is continuing reluctance to criticise the dominant economic model, even though it operates by destroying its own principal source of income (Andreff 2019). In order to justify perpetuating exploitation and inequality, the dominant neoliberal ideology has erected powerful, self-sustaining myths that are difficult to overcome (Shefner and Blad 2019). One of these myths is the idea that the best way to organise government-run public services is by turning them over to private organisations to run on behalf of the government.

Whether the government is running the services directly or paying another business to run them, if the service is necessary then the expense of running it remains. However, in order to gain more profit, the business may reduce the quality of the service by requiring staff to do more, but with restrictions on practice, less training or using poorer quality materials. The companies providing services then become an influence on the government by seeking opportunities to develop and expand their business in order to increase their profits, since their only customer is the government. These companies employ government employees as advisors who, in turn, are attractive as government employees because of their association with the business. A revolving door of influence develops, through which government increasingly comes under the influence of the organisations it employs and, instead of serving its population, serves the businesses it is employing (Wrenn 2016).

These ideas are embedded in a neoliberal consensus that the market is the best possible way to organise trade (see Chapter 2). They are backed by global values, which are exported as aspirational consumer goals by multinational corporations and unelected trade organisations to the poorer countries, which they can dominate through economic power. Although there has been a recent comment on this phenomenon as an effect of neoliberal global policy, it was previously a feature of colonial policy (Madeley 2009; Tharoor 2018).

Occupational therapy as a commodity

In some countries, these myths and goals have supported the introduction of occupational therapy as part of an exchange of values. While it served a humanitarian purpose, for example, in response to the poliomyelitis epidemic of the 1940s and 1950s, which affected many parts of the world and particularly Latin American countries, occupational therapy was also seen as an attractive technology. As an export from the Western economies, whose colonial policies had done much to shape Latin America's uneven development, occupational therapy offered aspirational opportunities to a rising middle class (or, at least, contributed to the emancipation of women in that socioeconomic group) and potentially reduced the economic dependency of people with disabilities by making them available to work (see Box 5.3).

Box 5.3   Exporting occupational therapy as a new health technology

Occupational therapy was introduced in Argentina through a group led by Mary MacDonald, in response to the 1950s poliomyelitis epidemic (Macdonald 1961; Monzeli, Morrison and Lopes 2019). In 1955, Argentina experienced a military coup that ousted the populist president, Juan Perón. In the following years, relations with the United States and the United Kingdom included a series of economic missions to the military government, following International Monetary Fund principles. Occupational therapy was offered to Argentina, along with trade contracts and car factories, as a technology that could address some of the pressing issues in the country, such as rehabilitation; both as a humanitarian aspect of public health systems, through cooperation between the World Health Organization and the Argentine and British governments, and in terms of enabling people with disabilities to work (Monzeli, Morrison and Lopes 2019). Occupational therapy was also an aspirational career for middle class, white women at a time of rising incomes and changing roles in parts of Latin American society.

Mary MacDonald was born in South America, to British parents, and by the early 1960s was the Principal of the Dorset House School of Occupational Therapy (Wilcock 2001). Her account of starting an occupational therapy training programme in Argentina (Macdonald 1961) made a passing reference to the Perón regime but did not mention the Western economic interests that formed part of the backdrop to her mission (Beaulac 1959; Galheigo 2011; Monzeli, Morrison and Lopes 2019).

Macdonald's (1961) experience, as the leader of a small band of occupational therapists setting up a training programme in an exotic location, is an almost parochial account; a personal narrative recounted for the British occupational therapy community. Viewed in terms of social practice theory, that experience was shaped by the teleoaffective structures formed by the nexus of the group's development grant, intergovernmental relations, Argentinian society and their own sense of what were appropriate responses to the situation they found. MacDonald and her colleagues established a performance of occupational therapy practice grounded in the practical realities of the circumstances of the mission she and her colleagues had been given.

Looking back, 60 years on, the establishment of the occupational therapy profession in Argentina can be judged successful, with journals and programmes located in different parts of the country. Furthermore, occupational therapists in Argentina have worked through significant challenges in maintaining a sense of identity as a profession that is sited in the global South, emancipated from its colonial origins and reflects social needs (Bottinelli et al. 2016).

Resisting social inequality

It can be difficult to conceptualise alternatives to the free market economy but there are other ideas about how people can exchange goods or resources and contribute work or effort. Some of these derive from societies without money, such as the Wiradjuri described in Chapter 3, where there might be a higher dependency on the environment. Such ideas, which are set out in utopian perspectives such as Morris's *News from Nowhere* (2002/1890), are sometimes dismissed as romantic nostalgia for the past. However, they can also be seen to represent pragmatic knowledge systems that influence social practices and allow people to live a sustainable existence in different natural environments (Datta 2015).

The social economist, Gill Seyfang (2006), a keen advocate of time banks, argued that the exchange of time as value is an 'occupational therapy' (p. 438) through which socially excluded people can use the asset of personal time for the reciprocal realisation of the benefits of active citizenship. Occupational therapists, working with social inclusion, health promotion and social prescribing projects around, for example, active ageing, may be involved in a variety of schemes that include alternative economic stratagems, such as time banks, repair cafes, skills exchanges, food banks and community gardens (Neary, Walker and Zaidi 2016; Momori and Richards 2017; Beagan, Chapman and Power 2018).

We began this section by conceptualising occupational therapy as *a constellation of practice*, in common with other healthcare professions. We then considered two of the wider social issues that provided the context for the emergence, development and future of the allied health professions: the legacy of colonialism and social inequality. For example, while the origins of occupational therapy and physiotherapy in Latin America may be linked to the global polio epidemic of the mid-20th century, social and political dimensions are also significant to their histories, such as the imperialism associated with the Cold War and post-colonial legacy (Monzeli, Morrison and Lopes 2019; Giraldo-Pedroza et al. 2021). Since the object of occupational therapy is largely around meaning and participation in occupation, as we saw in Chapter 2, the profession and its underpinning knowledge base must also recognise the wider context of social practices and the formation of constellations of practice.

The next section identifies some of the major social issues currently influencing the practice of occupational therapists around the world.

Global social issues

Some of the key social issues facing the world are linked to the legacy of colonialism and social structures of inequality, described above. The four issues discussed in this section are as follows: climate change, inequality, sustainability and human displacement.

Climate change

Current climate changes have been found to be related to human activity, including economic and industrial development (IPCC 2022). Human exploitation of natural resources for fuel, manufacturing and agriculture has resulted in significant global warming, at a rate that now threatens the viability of planetary ecosystems. The global economy, serving the interests of powerful corporations and dominant political forces, continues to drive demands that increase the effects of global warming. On the one hand, countries such as Australia, with huge, opencast coal mining operations, have been reluctant to support initiatives that reduce the consumption of fossil fuel; on the other hand, impoverished people clear forests for land to cultivate crops or build homes (Mensah 2019).

Climate change has a disproportionate impact on low- and middle-income countries, which not only experience greater changes than wealthier nations but have fewer resources to manage the consequences; such as comprehensive health services or early warning systems (WHO 2015; World Meteorological Organization 2021). Although death tolls from climate change events, such as droughts, have fallen in the last 50 years, the economic cost of climate change is significantly increasing with the frequency of weather events.

The cost of economic damage may seem more significant in wealthier countries, because of greater infrastructure and property value, but the impact is relative. Poorer countries and regions take longer to recover from disasters and deaths from natural disasters are higher in low- and middle-income countries. Climate incidents and processes are themselves complex; for example, a tropical cyclone may generate storm surges, flooding and heavy rain, and further complications may result from power outages or collapsed buildings. The example given in Box 5.4 illustrates this inequality.

Box 5.4   The unequal impact of climate change

One of the most vulnerable nations on the planet is the Republic of Kiribati, based in a group of coral atolls in the Pacific Ocean, most of which are about one or two metres above sea level. With the rising sea level caused by climate change, the decreasing amount of living space has concentrated the population in the capital, Tarawa, where overcrowding has affected the freshwater supply and spread disease.

It will be only a few decades before this island republic disappears, therefore the government is planning for the population to be resettled before this happens. A Kiribati man, Ioanne Teitiota, whose family was living temporarily in New Zealand, applied for refugee status on the basis of the threat presented by climate change. However, he failed to establish a basis for the persecution that would enable him to be defined as a refugee by the New Zealand government.

Although wealthy, industrialised nations have contributed disproportionately to climate change, no single organisation or government can be identified as directly responsible within an international legal system that reflects the power imbalance of the Global North versus Pacific island nations. Unless a plan is agreed upon for managed emigration due to climate change, the situation is likely to deteriorate into further refugee crises (Ni 2015).

Rising sea levels are not the only climate problem. Desertification creates numerous, complex effects; including contributing further to climate change, spreading invasive plant species and encouraging maladaptive intensive agricultural practices in many parts of the world (see, e.g., Brinkmann, Liehr and Bickel 2021). One effect of these pressures, for example, in the Sahel region of Africa, is that they generate inter-communal violence as people compete for increasingly scarce resources (Diop et al. 2018).

Inequity and health

One of the greatest threats to global health is the **inequity**, or lack of fairness of experience, found in every society, which arises through social **inequalities**, or differences in the conditions in which people live (Marmot 2017a, 2017b). An example of inequity in the United Kingdom is described in Box 5.5.

Box 5.5   Food inequity in a wealthy country

Inequity and precariousness impact people through the relationship between their material means and their access to health resources; not only healthcare but the very means of maintaining health, such as good food.

A study exploring the food shopping experiences of women on low incomes in the United Kingdom found that shopping to feed a family on a budget combines multiple, negative experiences (Beagan, Chapman and Power 2018). These experiences include feelings of shame, being the object of other people's snobbery, official accusations of irresponsibility, socially stigmatising moments of having to put items back because you cannot afford them and holding up checkout queues while counting change and coupons. Women described regularly living on peanut butter for a week, having periods when they could not afford to eat at all and queuing for hours at food banks to receive products that may be of little practical help. Furthermore, the women risked being unable to pay the rent or utility bills if they spent too much on food.

As the number of people experiencing food poverty in the United Kingdom has increased, professional rhetoric in public health and neoliberal government health policy have shifted the responsibility for health inequities from the State to those people who are undergoing the challenges of finding healthy foods for their families.

The experience of inequality operates through internalised oppression when less powerful people learn to perceive themselves as stigmatised and deserving of their circumstances because they are inferior. This internalisation of oppression was one of the intentions, and lasting consequences, of apartheid regimes and slavery (Luthuli 1962; Goffman 1963/1986; Linebaugh and Rediker 2001; Tyler and Slater 2018). Thus, macro economic policies that perpetuate inequality not only prefigure who has access to certain social practices but also set in train internal mechanisms that maintain people in positions of inferiority. For example, the United Nations has described homelessness as a result of

> government acquiescence to real estate speculation, a result of treating housing as a commodity rather than a human right. It is rooted in a global privileging of wealth and power, accompanied by blaming and scorning those who have little.
>
> (UN 2019: 1)

Inequality becomes economic violence 'where structural and systemic policy and political choices that are skewed in favor of the richest and most powerful people, result in direct harm to the vast majority of ordinary people worldwide' (Oxfam 2022: 12). Even where public institutions provide a range of services to social classes who are economically unable to provide for themselves, the effect is to sustain the social practices of survival with poverty. For example, many working people on low incomes, in countries of the Global North, can obtain very basic levels of social security (Shefner and Blad 2019). This, in turn, makes it possible for businesses to employ people on wages that would otherwise make their lives unsustainable. One example of this is the phenomenon of older people in the United States alternating between welfare and zero-hours contracted, low-paid jobs in global distribution company centres (https://hiring.amazon.com/our-team/camperforce#/), national parks and the agricultural sector (Bruder 2017).

Sustainability

The long-term social and economic effects of colonialism have prefigured a global demand for levelling up, in terms of life quality and consumer experience, in those countries where development capacity was sequestered or undermined (Tharoor 2018). However, the quantity of goods and the cost of lifestyles and technologies needed to achieve upwards equalisation could destroy the planet (Max-Neef 2010). Unsustainable demands for lifestyle goods far beyond sustenance, such as the cultivation of soya for cattle food to provide red meat for corporate suppliers, or the professional sponsorship of one elite athlete to wear sports clothes amounting to more than the wages of the entire workforce and the factory system producing them, have led to much of the planet becoming either urbanised or else under agricultural production; forming ecosystems that can be categorised as **anthropogenic biomes**. This term describes patterns of land use or human-environment interactions that result in altered ecosystems, such as dense urban settlements or agricultural croplands. These biomes form a mosaic over the planet's surface, consisting of areas of urbanisation, cultivation or remaining wilderness.

A series of maps, showing the changing nature of this mosaic of anthropogenic biomes, shows how wild areas have been progressively lost over the years since 1700 (https://sedac.ciesin.columbia.edu/data/collection/anthromes/sets/browse). Wilderness areas are complex ecosystems that are rapidly being eroded by human activity and even those wild areas that remain, such as the polar ice caps or the rainforests of the Indonesian archipelago, are affected, by environmental threats or climate change. These areas, whether on land or marine, are significant areas of biodiversity for potential carbon storage and retention through species interaction and soil retention. Once they are gone, the former degree of complexity that has been lost cannot be restored through processes such as reforestation (Soto-Navarro et al. 2020).

Human development does not only produce environmental changes that impact the climate and ecology. The development of human society and technological capability involves social practices that are associated with non-communicable and lifestyle diseases, such as obesity and auto-immune disease (Wolf 2015). Various social practices and their materialities are associated with particular patterns of consumption, such as the types and quantity of food eaten, tooth cleaning products used, tools employed in growing food or disposal of paint thinners after painting a door. Often, people are unaware that the resources they use, including the ingredients and packaging of food products, have environmental consequences (Wakefield-Rann, Fam and Stewart 2020). Many of the products employed in the practices of everyday life, such as house cleaning, are directly or indirectly harmful to both the wider environment and the person performing the practice. For example, bleach may not only kill pests and germs but also contaminate household surfaces, sewage systems and water tables. It can be difficult to eliminate these products, even after they have been shown to have adverse effects, because they are an integral part of domestic practices.

Sustainability is the responsibility of everyone and begins with what people do in their everyday lives (Ikiugu 2008; Mensah 2019). As we have seen in the climate change examples above, domestic activities carried out in one place have an impact on the habitats of people in others. Max-Neef (2010) outlined a development philosophy based on the satisfaction of human needs. He classified the basic requirements for development into nine categories: subsistence, protection, affection, understanding, participation, idleness, creation, identity and freedom, giving examples of how these needs can be satisfied. One of these satisfiers is a place to be, which includes both a physical space and a virtual space from which a person is able to interact and belong in the world. Max-Neef (2010) extended this concept from the micro-level, in literally having a space on this earth, to the macro-level of earth where there are spaces for people to be and within which they can engage in social practices.

Displacement

The fourth area of global concern is the increasing number of displaced people. These include refugees, fleeing from deteriorating political situations, migrants, driven from home by climate change emergencies and natural disasters, and economic migrants who wish to escape poverty and seek new opportunities. Unmet needs, created by factors such as youth unemployment and food price shocks, promote huge unrest and can result in population movements: both within countries and across national borders.

Within countries, people have historically migrated from the countryside to the cities, where goods, services, manufacturing and distribution centres are concentrated, along with the myriad jobs they provide. This happened, for example, with the growth of supercities in Brazil at the end of the 20th century and is part of the background to the development of social occupational therapy in that country (Lopes and Malfitano 2020). People may move between countries for their own and their families' safety, to improve their economic status or simply to earn enough money to support their families, as happened when oil prices collapsed in Venezuela during the 2010s (Durán and Cuevas 2020).

Currently, the occupational therapy profession, along with other health professions (Giraldo-Pedroza et al. 2021), is engaged in a process of exploring the broader realities that impact health needs and how they can be met. Although there is a tendency for English to dominate professional discourses, these realities traverse the borders of language, and also those of class, race and other intersectionalities. Some of these issues are explored in the next section.

Where the profession is now: A turning point?

This book developed from the editors' and authors' concerns about the capacity of the dominant theories and models employed in occupational therapy to guide the profession effectively through the choices we face globally and into a future that matches our aspirations. The profession is evidencing unease about our theoretical base, for example, in relation to the complexity of occupation as both a concept and the basis for intervention (Pentland et al. 2018); our understanding of socially sanctioned, or dark, occupations (Twinley 2021); the cultural basis of dominant occupational therapy theories and models (Hammell 2011, 2019; Reid 2020), and inherent racisms and exclusions (Ramugondo 2018; Grenier 2020).

This section considers the role that occupational therapy scholarship and theory might play in shaping the future of the profession as a constellation of practice. While recognising that the allied health professions have been, and continue to be, directed by the ideologies of biomedicine and neoliberal economics (Nicholls 2017), we propose that the development of integrated theories of occupation and occupational therapy, drawn from a broad range of intellectual and cultural perspectives, will clarify the social role of the profession and strengthen our professional identity.

Issues for occupational therapy

Some of the drivers of change in healthcare practices result from tensions, and even conflict, within institutional processes (Holland and Lave 2019). Like other allied health professions, in countries around the world, occupational therapy finds its work and orientation determined to a large extent by the demands of medicine and finance (amongst other influences, such as gender and race). For example, current UK policy on the integration of health and social care services tends to respond to the demands of powerful groups, such as doctors, and risks marginalising those professions that are smaller in number. The limits to professional autonomy, consequent on such marginalisation, restrict our capacity to articulate the relevance of occupational therapy for particular roles (Walder et al. 2021).

The health and social care policy trajectory in Europe, for example, strongly suggests a shift towards primary care, which is most likely to be led by the medical and nursing professions, but there are challenges due to politicians' lack of understanding of rehabilitation services. Some of the key issues were identified by Bolt and colleagues (2019) and Spiess et al. (2021):

- The proportion of occupational therapists working in primary care is low compared to those working in other services, even in countries with relatively strong primary care systems, such as the United Kingdom or the Netherlands.
- The capacity of education and training systems to produce a sufficient supply of people to fill additional primary care posts may be inadequate, and many countries have much lower numbers of occupational therapists than others in relation to their populations.
- Where occupational therapists are allocated to primary care settings, there are often insufficient numbers, working single-handed and carrying unrealistic case loads; with little understanding of their role from other professionals, politicians and the general public.

These issues act in combination with the narrow demographic profile in the occupational therapy workforce and are reinforced by patriarchal and medical dominance (Bottinelli et al. 2016; Orton 2021). Occupational therapists have to be critically aware of wider social and political realities, and of the relationship between the activities they might propose to negotiate with people and the historical and temporal context of those activities. At the same time, occupational therapists have to communicate the nature and purpose of their work with fellow professionals and other actors in the field, while remaining flexible enough to allow their practice to be shaped around both individual and community needs.

Alternative approaches to the biomedical model of healthcare include the one health model, developed in the Global South. In the **one health model**, all health is regarded as part of a single, interactive system; from the health of individual creatures to that of the entire planet (Davis and Sharp 2020). However, there is a risk that such approaches can, if taken up by a medical hierarchy, become oversimplified. For example, a focus on the disease aspects of cross-species contamination, such as bird flu and COVID-19, ignores the socioeconomic and environmental factors that bring large numbers of people and animals into close, physical contact (Hinchliffe 2015).

Within the occupational therapy profession, there is a growing concern with social transformation, which could be seen as something of a return to the reformist project described in Chapter 1 (Farias et al. 2018; Rudman et al. 2018; Cunningham et al. 2020). **Social transformation** is about producing positive changes in society through activism. **Activism** involves social practices based on collaboration and collectivity, where individuals can work out their own solutions and identify the changes needed (Holland and Lave 2019) by working against common problems. For occupational therapists, this is in contrast to a routinised *praktik* of diagnosis, formulation and treatment.

However, many of the approaches developed by occupational therapists to bring about social transformation are challenging professional practice in the global North because of how occupational therapy services are shaped, within both state and private healthcare systems. For most of the people occupational therapists work with around the world, the common problems are not diseases but the economic, political, environmental and social situations that promote disease (Marmot 2020).

Recognition of these issues, and the part that occupational therapists might play in maintaining an unequal status quo through their position in a hegemony (Nancarrow and Borthwick 2021), has also contributed to unease about the project of occupational therapy being limited by its co-location with certain other social practices (Orton 2021). For example, occupational therapists working in multidisciplinary teams may find themselves adopting the meanings and competences of the team, rather than employing profession-specific goals and skills or finding some form of compromise through which they can strive to demonstrate the value of their professional practice.

The pattern of occupational therapy as an exported social practice has already been mentioned (see Box 5.3); in many countries, practitioners are coming to question the relevance of values and theories that were devised within the culture of wealthy and colonial societies (Ramugondo 2018; White and Beagan 2020; Murthi and Hammell 2021). This work requires a scholarly activism in which people reach out and engage with the literature and scholarship of others. The construction of a stronger theoretical framework for occupational therapy depends on this but, since people outside the anglosphere have had to work through the medium of English, there is a real need for anglophones to address their lack of fluency in other languages. Scholarship cannot continue only on the basis of what is available in English, to the exclusion and obliteration of other perspectives that are not accessible to those in the most powerful positions, because they cannot read them.

Theory: An element of the social practice of occupational therapy

In the context of this chapter, the term **scholarship** is used to refer to the development and organisation of occupational therapy knowledge through study and research (Shorter Oxford English Dictionary 2002). A **scholar** is a person who advances or refines the knowledge base of occupational therapy.

The knowledge base of occupational therapy consists of concepts and theories that are organised in ways that support the practitioner's clinical and professional reasoning. A **concept** is 'a principle of classification ... that can guide us in determining whether an entity belongs in a given class' (Audi 1999: 170). Concepts, and their classification, are agreed within a particular community, such as a language group, a profession or a scholarly discipline, and are given names by which the community can refer to them. Examples of concepts used in the occupational therapy community include *activities of daily living*, *occupational performance*, *activity analysis* and *functional assessment*.

Concepts are the building blocks of theory (Creek 2014); hence, occupational therapy theories are constructed from the core concepts of the profession. A **theory** is a conceptual system or framework used to organise knowledge in order to understand or shape reality (Bryant, Fieldhouse and Bannigan 2014: 485). Occupational therapists use theories to help them to 'understand cause and effect and to make predictions about the likely outcomes of intervention, so that the most appropriate and effective course of action can be undertaken' (Creek 2014: 34). An example of an occupational therapy theory is Wilcock's occupational theory of human nature (Wilcock 2006), which explains the relationship between health and occupation. Models such as the Model of Human Occupation (Kielhofner and Burke 1980) or the Canadian Occupational Performance Model (Law et al. 1990) are significant ideas in the theory of occupational therapy, which serve to explain how individuals engage in occupations. As therapists and researchers develop experiments and projects to provide evidence that people function in the ways outlined by these models, they increasingly become incorporated into professional practice and understandings of the nature of occupation.

Theory is thus an element of the constellation of practice that is occupational therapy. According to Shove and colleagues (2012), the three elements of a social practice are materials, competences and meanings. Within this classification, **meaning** is 'the social and symbolic significance of participation [in a practice] at any one moment' (Shove et al. 2012: 23). For the occupational therapy practitioner, the significance of participation in occupational therapy is linked to the profession's purpose, goals, values and social status, and to the practitioner's identity, motivation and affect during a given performance. Theory contributes to the meaning that occupational therapy has for practitioners and others, through its framing of the purpose, goals and methods of practice; for example, Wilcock's occupational theory of human nature suggests a strong role for occupational therapists in the 'research and development of population health approaches that take an occupational perspective' (2006: 211).

When we view occupational therapy as a social practice, therefore, it is apparent that working to extend, deepen and rationalise our professional knowledge base will help to clarify our purpose, strengthen our identity, enhance our confidence and justify our interventions. This is particularly important when the professional goals of occupational therapists diverge from those of the organisations that employ them, as explored in Chapter 2.

In order for occupational therapy to continue developing as a profession, we need to adopt wider and more critical perspectives than those offered by biomedicine and neoliberal economics. We have already set out, in the sections above, some of the global issues that impact health, and have identified the need to connect with knowledge frameworks from other languages than the dominant anglosphere. The concept of occupation, encompassing a full range of human activity, could be too large and complex to encapsulate in a discipline. However, to overlook or ignore perspectives that may illuminate how people do, be, belong and become would be to miss issues that may have a complex relationship with healthy outcomes. In the narrow social profile that has characterised the occupational therapy profession for many years, previously neglected areas, such as influences from the global south and black or feminist scholarship, have the potential to provide broader understandings of the different times and spaces (Grenier 2020) in which occupational therapies and social practices may be understood (see Chapter 9).

Emergent practices challenge theoretical models and clinical approaches based on medical tradition. They demand bespoke interventions that, to be effective, have to be informed by the context of culture, class and society.

Emerging practice

A term that is often used in connection with community development and innovative approaches to occupational therapy is *emerging practice*. However, much of what is now described as 'emerging' has antecedents stretching back through the history of the profession and may represent everyday practice in some parts of the world (Alers and Crouch 2010; Thew et al. 2012). The historical, colonial developments of the last 200 years have been instrumental in providing the context for the expansion of occupational therapy in the latter half of the 20th century, particularly in countries under British or American economic and political influence. These conditions made it possible to export occupational therapy as a new health technology, with countries encouraged to take up the profession in their developing health systems (see Box 5.3).

The occupational therapy mantra of *doing, being, becoming and belonging* (Wilcock 1998; Hitch, Pépin and Stagnitti 2014) implies a narrative of occupation that includes not merely individual, lived time, as explored in Chapter 3. The expression of doing, being, becoming and belonging is reciprocated through interaction with other people and communities and, by extension, also intergenerational practice-as-entity. This conceptualisation of occupation suggests a trajectory in which occupations might be inherited and passed on, along which it might be possible to collaborate on action to deflect performances away from negative outcomes and towards positive goals. Examples of such action, discussed above, include social activism, through community members developing a local project to create a resource such as a park; or the activism of the Futurians, in supporting what became a global popular literary genre, enjoyed and participated in by millions of people.

Such a trajectory is not reducible to a clinical process because it is embedded in a nexus of social, historical, cultural and economic practices and is shaped by environments and spaces. As described in Chapter 3, social practices are entities in space and time and, as such, are not reducible to repeatable components. Indeed, each time a practice is performed, it leads to a slightly different outcome, as all practices evolve and are honed through repetition by different performers in different contexts.

These expanded dimensions of occupation and occupational therapy are recognised in some of those countries where the profession is most challenged, by socioeconomic divisions, to make an effective difference to life quality. These divisions are often encountered at the points where societies are most diverse and where minority communities are at risk of being marginalised or even rendered invisible (see Box 5.6).

Box 5.6   Social occupational therapy

Social occupational therapy (Lopes and Malfitano 2020) grew out of late 20th-century political changes in Brazil, as it transitioned from a military dictatorship to a democracy. Brazilian occupational therapy training had an uncertain history, from its origins in the 1950s until the need for the profession was more widely recognised in the 1970s (Reis and Lopes 2018). As the first trainees began to seek post-graduate qualifications, they had to resort to programmes in psychology, sociology and anthropology, because none was available in occupational therapy. Applying their new knowledge to the profession opened up the possibility of a socially engaged profession, initially sited in the university departments where the subject was taught, working around the extreme conditions of poverty found in the favelas in the megacities of Southern Brazil.

In this section, we have seen that, while occupational therapy is a relatively small and powerless profession in the fields of health and social care, it has qualities and practices that are relevant to current global needs. Some of the strengths of the profession have been identified: the increasing diversity of the global workforce, the activist roots of occupational therapy and emerging areas of occupational therapy practice outside mainstream services.

Summary and conclusion

This chapter began with a summary of the historical development of the occupational therapy profession, as described in the first part of this book. It highlighted how some of the social and contextual influences on that development, including colonialism and embedded social inequality, have left the profession with a legacy that needs to be critically unpicked if occupational therapy is to remain relevant and valued in the modern world. The central section of the chapter identified some of the global social issues with which occupational therapists need to engage in revisiting, and possibly redefining, their social role and purpose.

The chapter finished with an overview of where the occupational therapy profession is now, in terms of the key social and professional issues it faces, the current state of occupational therapy scholarship and emerging areas of practice.

In the second part of the book, in Chapters 6, 7 and 8, we consider in more depth how occupational therapists are responding to the challenges facing the profession. These responses are addressed in three categories: access, resources and change.

References

Alers, V., and Crouch, R. (eds.) (2010) *Occupational therapy: an african perspective.* Cape Town: Sara Shorten.

Andreff, W. (2019) The unintended emergence of a greed-led economic system. *Kybernetes,* 48(2): 238–252. 10.1108/K-01-2018-0018

Asimov, I. (1980). *Memory yet green: the autobiography of Isaac Asimov, 1920–1954.* New York: Avon Books.

Audi, R. (1999). *Cambridge dictionary of philosophy,* 2nd ed. Cambridge: Cambridge University Press.

Beagan, B.L., Chapman, G.E., and Power, E. (2018) The visible and invisible occupations of food provisioning in low income families. *Journal of Occupational Science,* 25(1): 100–111.

Beaulac, W.L. (1959) The situation in Argentina. Foreign relations of the United states, 1958–1960, American Republics, Volume V. Document 199. https://history.state.gov/historicaldocuments/frus1958-60v05/d199

Black, J. (2018) The United Kingdom and British empire: a figurational approach. *Rethinking History,* 22(1): 3–24.

Bolt, M., Ikking, T., Baaijen, R., and Saenger, S. (2019) Occupational therapy and primary care. *Primary Health Care Research and Development,* 20: e27. 10.1017/S1463423618000452

Bottinelli, M.M., Nabergoi, M., Mattei, M.C., Zorzoli, F.J.M., Díaz, F.M., Spallato, N.M., Mulholland, M., Bredereke, M.M.M.D.P., Sartirana, A.M.G., Briglia, J., and Daneri, S.M. (2016) Reflexiones sobre los orígenes de la formación en Terapia Ocupacional en Argentina. *Revista Ocupación Humana,* 16(2): 11–25.

Brinkmann, K., Liehr, S., and Bickel, L. (2021) Rangeland management in Namibia in the face of Looming desertification: Insights from the freehold Farmers' perspective. XXIV international grassland congress/XI international rangeland congress (sustainable use of grassland and rangeland resources for Improved livelihoods). Kenya agricultural and livestock research organization. Online at https://uknowledge.uky.edu/igc/24/5/1/. Accessed May 2022.

Bruder, J. (2017) *Nomadland: surviving America in the twenty-first century.* New York, NY: Norton.

Bryant, W., Fieldhouse, J., and Bannigan, K. (eds.) (2014) *Creek's occupational therapy and mental health,* 5th ed. Edinburgh: Churchill Livingstone Elsevier.

Creek, J. (2014) The knowledge base of occupational therapy. In: W. Bryant, J. Fieldhouse and K. Bannigan (eds.) *Creek's occupational therapy and mental health,* 5th ed. Edinburgh: Churchill Livingstone Elsevier. 27–47.

Cunningham, M., Warren, A., Pollard, N., and Abey, S. (2020) Enacting social transformation through occupation: a narrative literature review. *Scandinavian Journal of Occupational Therapy,* 1–20. https://www.tandfonline.com/doi/full/10.1080/11038128.2020.1841287

Datta, R. (2015) A relational theoretical framework and meanings of land, nature, and sustainability for research with indigenous communities. *Local Environment,* 20(1): 102–113.

Davis, A., and Sharp, J. (2020). Rethinking one health: emergent human, animal and environmental assemblages. *Social Science and Medicine,* 258: 113093. 10.1016/j.socscimed.2020.113093

der Merwe, V., and Rauch, T. (2019) *The political construction of occupational therapy in South Africa: critical analysis of a curriculum as discourse* (Doctoral dissertation, University of the Free State).

Diop, S., Guisse, A., Sene, C., Cisse, B., Diop, N.R., Ka, S.D., ... and Yongdong, W. (2018). Combating desertification and improving local livelihoods through the GGWI in the Sahel region: the example of Senegal. *Journal of Resources and Ecology*, 9(3): 257–265.

Durán, M.G. , and Cuevas, D. (2020) Colombia-Venezuela: the humanitarian crisis of the Venezuelan migration flow. In: A.A. Mateos, M.G. Durán, C.E. Villaseñor and J.I. Martínez (eds.) *Migratory flows at the borders of our world*. Bogota: Editorial Pontificia Universidad Javeriana. 249–274.

Farias, L., Laliberte Rudman, D., Pollard, N., Schiller, S., Serrata Malfitano, A.P., Thomas, K., and Bruggen, H.V. (2018) Critical dialogical approach: a methodological direction for occupation-based social transformative work. *Scandinavian Journal of Occupational Therapy.* 10.1080/11038128.2018.1469666

Flinders, M. (2021) Democracy and the politics of coronavirus: trust, blame and understanding. *Parliamentary Affairs*, 74(2): 483–502. ISSN 0031-2290. 10.1093/pa/gsaa013

Galheigo, S.M. (2011) Occupational therapy in the social field: concepts and critical considerations. In: F. Kronenberg, N. Pollard and D. Sakellariou (eds.) *Occupational therapies without borders: towards an ecology of occupation-based practices (Volume 2)*. Edinburgh: Elsevier Science. 47–56.

Giraldo-Pedroza, A., Robayo-Torres, A.L., Guerrero, A.V.S., and Nicholls, D.A. (2021) Narrative histories of physiotherapy in Colombia, Ecuador, and Argentina. *Physiotherapy Theory and Practice*, 37(3): 447–459.

Goffman, E. (1986/1963) *Stigma: notes on the management of spoiled identity*. New York, NY: Simon and Schuster.

Grenier, M.L. (2020) Cultural competency and the reproduction of white supremacy in occupational therapy education. *Health Education Journal*, 79(6): 633–644.

Hammell, K.W. (2011) Resisting theoretical imperialism in the disciplines of occupational science and occupational therapy. *British Journal of Occupational Therapy*, 74(1): 27–33.

Hammell, K.W. (2019) Building globally relevant occupational therapy from the strength of our diversity. *World Federation of Occupational Therapists Bulletin*, 75(1): 13–26.

Hickman, M.J., and Ryan, L. (2020) The "Irish question": marginalizations at the nexus of sociology of migration and ethnic and racial studies in Britain. *Ethnic and Racial Studies*, 43(16): 96–114.

Hinchliffe, S. (2015) More than one world, more than one health: re-configuring Interspecies health. *Social Science and Medicine*, 129: 28–35.

Hitch, D., Pépin, G., and Stagnitti, K. (2014) In the footsteps of Wilcock, part one: The evolution of doing, being, becoming, and belonging. *Occupational Therapy in Health Care*, 28(3): 231–246. 10.3109/07380577.2014.898114

Holland, D., and Lave, J. (2019) Social practice theory and the historical production of persons. In *Cultural-Historical Approaches to Studying Learning and Development*. Singapore: Springer. 235–248

Ikiugu, M.N. (2008) *Occupational science in the service of Gaia*. Baltimore, MD: PublishAmerica.

Intergovernmental Panel on Climate Change (2022) *Climate change 2022*. Online at https://www.ipcc.ch/report/sixth-assessment-report-cycle/. Accessed February 2022.

Jones, M. (2007) *Feast*. Oxford: Oxford University Press.

Joubert, R. (2010) Exploring the history of occupational therapy's development in South Africa to reveal the flaws in our knowledge base. *South African Journal of Occupational Therapy*, 40(3): 21–26.

Kenny, K. (2017) Irish emigrations in a comparative perspective. In E. Biagini and M. Daly (eds.) *The Cambridge social history of modern Ireland*. Cambridge: Cambridge University Press. 405.

Kielhofner, G., and Burke, J.P. (1980) A model of human occupation, part 1: Conceptual framework and content. *The American Journal of Occupational Therapy*, 34(9): 572–581.

Knight, D. (1977) *The futurians: the story of the science fiction "family" of the 30's that produced today's top SF writers and editors.* New York: John Day.

Lave, J., and Wenger, E. (1991) *Situated learning: legitimate peripheral participation.* Cambridge: Cambridge University Press.

Law, M., Baptiste, S., McColl, M., Opzoomer, A., Polatajko, H., and Pollock, N. (1990) The Canadian occupational performance measure: an outcome measure for occupational therapy. *Canadian Journal of Occupational Therapy*, 57(2): 82–87.

Linebaugh, P., and Rediker, M. (2001) *The many-headed hydra: sailors, slaves, commoners, and the hidden history of the revolutionary Atlantic.* London: Verso.

Lopes R., and Malfitano A. (eds.) (2020) *Social occupational therapy.* Edinburgh: Elsevier.

Luthuli A.J. (1962) *Let my people go.* London: Collins.

Macdonald, E.M. (1961) The responsibility of exporting a profession—opening an occupational therapy training school in the argentine. *Occupational Therapy: The Official Journal of the Association of Occupational Therapists*, 24(6): 14–19.

McLynn, F. (2011) *Napoleon.* Random House.

Madeley, J. (2009) *Big business, poor peoples: how transnational corporations damage the world's poor.* Chicago: Bloomsbury Publishing.

Marmot, M. (2017a) Social justice, epidemiology and health inequalities. *European Journal of Epidemiology*, 32(7): 537–546.

Marmot, M. (2017b) The health gap: the challenge of an unequal world: the argument. *International Journal of Epidemiology*, 46(4): 1312–1318.

Marmot, M. (2020) Health equity in England: the marmot review 10 years on. *British Medical Journal*, 368. 10.1136/bmj.m693

Max-Neef, M. (2010) The world on a collision course and the need for a new economy. *Ambio*, 39(3): 200–210.

Mensah, J. (2019) Sustainable development: meaning, history, principles, pillars, and implications for human action: literature review. *Cogent Social Sciences*, 5(1): 1653531. 10.1080/23311886.2019.1653531

Momori, N., and Richards, G. (2017) Service user and carer involvement: co-production. In: C. Long, J. Cronin-Davis and D. Cotterill (eds.) *Occupational therapy evidence in practice for mental health.* Chichester: Wiley. 17–34.

Montag, W. (2005) Necro-economics: Adam Smith and death in the life of the universal. *Radical Philosophy*, 134. https://www.radicalphilosophy.com/article/necro-economics

Monzeli, G.A., Morrison, R., and Lopes, R.E. (2019). Histories of occupational therapy in · Latin America: the first decade of creation of the education programs. *Cadernos Brasileiros de Terapia Ocupacional*, 27: 235–250.

Morris, W. (2002/1890) *News from nowhere.* Peterborough, Ontario: Broadview Press.

Murthi, K., and Hammell, K.W. (2021) Choice' in occupational therapy theory: a critique from the situation of patriarchy in India. *Scandinavian Journal of Occupational Therapy*, 28(1): 1–12.

Nancarrow, S., and Borthwick, A. (2021) *The allied health professions: a sociological perspective.* Bristol: Policy Press.

Neary, D., Walker, A., and Zaidi, A. (2016) A major report synthesising knowledge on active ageing in Europe. Sheffield, Mobilising the potential of active ageing in Europe (MoPAct). http://mopact.group.shef.ac.uk/wp-content/uploads/2013/10/D1.2-Synthesis-report-active-ageing-in-Europe.pdf

Ni, X.Y. (2015) A nation going under: legal protection for climate change refugees. *Boston College International and Comparative Law Review*, 38: 329. https://heinonline.org/HOL/Page?collection=journalsandhandle=hein.journals/bcic38andid=336andmen_tab=srchresults

Nicholls, D.A. (2017) *The end of physiotherapy.* Abingdon: Routledge.

Obregon, L. (2018). Empire, racial capitalism and international law: the case of manumitted Haiti and the recognition debt. *Leiden Journal of International Law*, 31(3): 597–615.

Orton, Y.T. (2021) *"A fine race of girls": occupational therapy and clinical governance in the district health boards of Aotearoa New Zealand* (Doctoral dissertation, Auckland University of Technology). https://openrepository.aut.ac.nz/handle/10292/14745

Oxfam (2022) *Inequality kills: Oxfam briefing paper*. Online at https://oxfamilibrary. openrepository.com/bitstream/handle/10546/621341/bp-inequality-kills-170122-en.pdf. Accessed January 2022.

Pentland, D., Kantartzis, S., Clausen, M.G., and Witemyre, K. (2018) *Occupational therapy and complexity: defining and describing practice*. London: Royal College of Occupational Therapists.

Perryman-Fox, M., and Cox, D.L. (2020) Occupational therapy in the United Kingdom: past, present, and future. *Annals of International Occupational Therapy*, 1(3): 144–151.

Peters, C.O. (2011) Powerful occupational therapists: a community of professionals, 1950–1980. *Occupational Therapy in Mental Health*, 27(3–4): 199–410.

Peters, C., Martin, P., and Mahoney, W. (2015) The power of two: Willard and Spackman's influence on occupational therapy. *American Journal of Occupational Therapy*, 69 (Supplement_1), 6911510215p1–6911510215p1.

Pollard, N., Kelly, S., Harrop, D., Flower, E., Dearns, M., Chan, M., Afzal, M., Munton, D., Perry-Young, L., Severn, A., Edler, R., Hills, E., Dubinko, N., and Woodward, A. (2020) *A report on the contemporary assessment of occupational therapy research in the UK. Project Report*. London/Sheffield, Royal College of Occupational Therapists/Sheffield Hallam University. http://shura.shu.ac.uk/27707/

Ramugondo, E. (2018) Healing work: intersections for decoloniality. *World Federation of Occupational Therapists Bulletin*, 74(2): 83–91.

Reid, H. (2020). *The rise (and suggested demise) of occupation-based models of practice* (Doctoral dissertation, Auckland University of Technology).

Reis, S.C.C.A.G., and Lopes, R.E. (2018) The beginning of the trajectory of occupational therapy academic institutionalization in Brazil: what pioneer professors tell about the creation of the first courses. *Cadernos Brasileiros de Terapia Ocupacional*, 26: 255–270.

Rudman, D.L., Pollard, N., Craig, C., Kantartzis, S., Piskur, B., Simó, S., van Bruggen, H., and Schiller, S. (2018) Contributing to social transformation through occupation. Experiences from a think tank. *Journal of Occupational Science*. 10.1080/14427591.2018.1538898

Seyfang, G. (2006) Harnessing the potential of the social economy? Time banks and UK public policy. *International Journal of Sociology and Social Policy*, 26(9/10): 430–443. 10.1108/ 01443330610690569

Shefner, J., and Blad, C. (2019) *Why austerity persists*. Cambridge: John Wiley and Sons.

Shorter Oxford English Dictionary (2002) *Shorter Oxford English Dictionary*. Oxford: Oxford University Press.

Shove, E., Pantzar, M. , and Watson, M. (2012) *The dynamics of social practice: everyday life and how it changes*. London: Sage.

Soto-Navarro, C., Ravilious, C., Arnell, A., De Lamo, X., Harfoot, M., Hill, S.L.L., … and Kapos, V. (2020) Mapping co-benefits for carbon storage and biodiversity to inform conservation policy and action. *Philosophical Transactions of the Royal Society* B, 375(1794): 20190128. 10.1098/rstb.2019.0128

Spiess, A.A.F., Skempes, D., Bickenbach, J., and Stucki, G. (2021) Exploration of current challenges in rehabilitation from the perspective of healthcare professionals: Switzerland as a case in point. *Health Policy*. 10.1016/j.healthpol.2021.09.010

Tharoor, S. (2018) *Inglorious empire: what the British did to India*. London: Penguin UK.

Thew, M., Edwards, M., Baptiste, S., and Molineux, M. (eds.) (2012) *Role emerging occupational therapy: maximising occupation focused practice*. Oxford: Wiley-Blackwell.

Twinley, R. (ed.) (2020) *Illuminating the dark side of occupation: international perspectives from occupational therapy and occupational science*. Abingdon: Routledge.

Tyler, I., and Slater, T. (2018) Rethinking the sociology of stigma. *The Sociological Review*, 66(4): 721–743. 10.1177/0038026118777425

United Nations (2019) 57th Session of the Commission for Social Development "Addressing inequalities and challenges to social inclusion through fiscal, wage and social protection policies" Homelessness: A Prominent Sign of Social Inequalities. https://www.un.org/development/desa/dspd/wp-content/uploads/sites/22/2019/02/Ireland_Homelessness-A-Prominent-Sign-of-Social-Inequalities-on-11-February-1.pdf

Varoufakis, Y. (2016) *And the weak suffer what they must?: Europe, austerity and the threat to global stability*. London: Penguin.

Wakefield-Rann, R., Fam, D., and Stewart, S. (2020) Routine exposure: social practices and environmental health risks in the home. *Social Theory and Health*, 18(4): 299–316.

Walder, K., Bissett, M., Molineux, M., and Whiteford, G. (2021) Understanding professional identity in occupational therapy: a scoping review. *Scandinavian Journal of Occupational Therapy*, 29(3): 1–23.

Wenger, E. (1998) *Communities of practice: learning, meaning and identity*. Cambridge: Cambridge University Press.

White, T., and Beagan, B.L. (2020) Occupational therapy roles in an indigenous context: an integrative review. *Canadian Journal of Occupational Therapy*, 87(3): 200–210.

Wilcock, A.A. (1998) *An occupational perspective of health*. Thorofare, NJ: Slack.

Wilcock, A.A. (2001) *Occupation for health: a journey from self health to prescription. Volume 2*. London: British Association and College of Occupational Therapists.

Wilcock, A.A. (2006) *An occupational perspective of health*, 2nd ed. Thorofare, NJ: Slack.

Wolf, M. (2015) Is there really such a thing as "one health"? Thinking about a more than human world from the perspective of cultural anthropology. *Social Science and Medicine*, 129: 5–11.

World Health Organization (WHO) (2015) *Human health and climate change in Pacific island countries*. Manila, Philippines: World Health Organization, Regional Office for the Western Pacific. Online at https://www.who.int/publications/i/item/human-health-and-climate-change-in-pacific-island-countries. Accessed May 2022.

World Meteorological Organization (2021) *WMO atlas of mortality and economic losses from weather, climate and water extremes (1970–2019)*. Geneva: WMO. Online at https://library.wmo.int/doc_num.php?explnum_id=10902. Accessed May 2022.

Wrenn, M.V. (2016) Immanent critique, enabling myths, and the neoliberal narrative. *Review of Radical Political Economics*, 48(3): 452–466.

6 Access

Elly Badcock, Elise Bromann Bukhave, and Jennifer Creek

Introduction

Each profession has a domain of concern that is 'essentially a statement of what the profession believes to be its area of expertise' (Mosey 1986: 7). The domain of concern of occupational therapy is occupation, in all its complexity and diversity, and what it means for people to be occupational beings. This chapter focuses on one aspect of occupation, access: how we understand access, why access to occupations is important, the barriers to access faced by different groups and ways of overcoming these barriers. It also addresses the issue of access to occupational therapy services.

To facilitate our understanding of issues of access, and how they relate both to occupational therapy and to health and social care more broadly, this chapter explores three distinct aspects of access (or the lack of it). The first section explores the myriad ways in which disabled people are denied access to the activities of daily living that form the focus of occupational therapy as a profession, from personal care to politics, and how these barriers to access are reflected and reproduced in health and social care services. The second section looks at how the structure of health and social care systems can act to deny access to services to disabled people and other marginalised groups. The third section looks more closely at how occupational therapists work with their clients on issues of access.

Occupational therapy and issues of access

Access is 'a way or means of approach or entrance' (Shorter Oxford English Dictionary 2002). This can refer to approaching or entering many different entities, for example, a physical environment, such as a building; a social environment, such as an educational programme; a resource, such as primary healthcare; a necessary condition for life, such as food; information, such as how to apply for benefits and facilities, such as transport. Occupational therapists are concerned with enabling access to any or all of these entities; not as an end in itself but as a means to enable occupation (Whybrow and Bridge 2015). Occupations can be seen as taking place within and being influenced by **social structures**, which are the ways that social relationships are ordered. Examples of social structures include social categories, such as students, regulations, such as criminal law and systems of symbolic communication, such as writing (Form and Wilterdink, n.d.).

DOI: 10.4324/9781003016755-6

Practice theorists take a different view of the relationship between how society is organised and what people do. From a practice theory perspective, social structures do not shape what people do but are created by the seemingly mundane practices that people engage in every day; these structures continue to exist only as long as daily practices keep being performed:

> A social world exists because of participants' unending and diverse work of reproducing and changing it … Though social structure is far from always at its participants' command, it is not external to social practice but a structural ordering of ongoing social practices.
>
> (Dreier 2008: 22)

Why is social structure relevant to the topic of access? Questions of access can be understood as huge political questions that have to be understood and changed on a grand scale, through policy, law and large-scale social consciousness campaigns. While this is important, trying to understand questions of access on only a macro-level means that we do not fully understand what access looks like for people who do not have it, or how barriers to access are maintained. Social practice theory allows us both to understand the social and historical context of the practices of everyday life and to zoom in to a micro-level and explore the everyday practices that keep society functioning. For example, the worker goes to work regularly for many reasons; from the social expectation that they will be productively employed, to material questions of where factories are built (for example, Amazon warehouses are located in Welsh ex-mining towns because of easy access to cheap labour), to individual, quotidian habits of time use.

This section explores issues of access from an occupational therapy perspective, using practice theory to frame the various issues. It begins with the different ways in which we might think about access, from physical movement in space to social participation. These understandings are then applied to issues of access in everyday life.

Alternative understandings of access

The term **access** is often understood as the ability to enter and move around physical buildings, facilities and transport (Sawyer and Bright 2014; Oxford Dictionary of Health and Social Care 2012). Indeed, access in this sense has for decades been a key focus for disability rights campaigns and social policy; from American wheelchair users crawling up the steps of the White House to demand accessible buildings (Welch 1990) to disabled people in the United Kingdom campaigning for properly accessible public toilets (Changing Places 2020). These inspiring campaigns around physical access are a necessary part of creating a society that can truly be said to be accessible, yet access means more than physical modifications to the built environment. Even if every necessary physical modification was made tomorrow, it is probable that other barriers to access would continue. For example, it is likely that people with noticeable facial differences would still be considered less attractive, employable and sociable (Stone and Wright 2013; Jamrozik et al. 2019); people with mental illness would still be under-employed, regardless of their qualifications (Trade Union Congress 2017), and people with learning disabilities would still die at a far younger age than those without learning disabilities (see Box 6.1).

Box 6.1   The impact of barriers to access

One group of people who face many barriers to access are those with learning disabilities, who experience large disparities in the quality of care they receive compared to people without learning disabilities. They are more likely to die in hospital, die or be seriously injured as a result of abuse or neglect, have serious illnesses that go undiagnosed and have their expressions of pain ignored (Regnard et al. 2003; Thornton 2019). In many cases, this disparity arises because healthcare professionals are not able to facilitate communication, due to a lack of understanding of learning disability (Morton-Nance and Schafer 2012; MENCAP 2018). There may be a Learning Disability Liaison Nurse, who can support other professionals, but they are likely to be stretched across an enormous caseload and have few resources (Stephenson 2018). The responsibility for the care of people with learning disabilities in hospitals, such as feeding, cleaning and administering medication, is often left with paid support workers or families (MENCAP 2012), regardless of whether they are equipped to provide this type of care. This leads to poorer health outcomes through a higher risk of infection, illness and death, and is another barrier to accessing appropriate healthcare.

People who have limited access to social and physical resources are described as **marginalised**. To be marginalised is 'to be different, excluded, unequal and potentially subjected to material deprivation or even extermination' (Duncan and Creek 2014: 461). People are marginalised on the basis of perceived differences, such as gender, race, social class, religion, sexual identity and physical disability. Box 6.2 explores disability as a social construction of difference.

Box 6.2   Disability perspective

Inequalities exist because disability is a social phenomenon quite distinct from the differences or impairments, physical or otherwise, that disabled people embody:

> In our view, it is society which disables physically impaired people. Disability is something imposed on top of our impairments, by the way we are unnecessarily isolated and excluded from full participation in society.
>
> (Barnes, Mercer and Shakespeare 2010)

Campaigns by the Union of Physically Impaired Against Segregation (UPIAS), in the United Kingdom, focused heavily on physical modifications to allow disabled people to partake fully in society, but they also highlighted a much wider issue; that disability is a product of society rather than of nature, and that questions of access must also focus on the social and cultural practices that work together to constitute disability. From this perspective, disability is not viewed as a feature of the individual but as 'representative of the cultural environment in which and through which our lives as embodied beings always appear' (Titchkosky 2008: 38).

Finding answers to difficult questions around access, health and disability necessitates delving into a troubling history of exclusion: the formative era of medically studying and treating disability is impossible to separate from the era of eugenics and the atrocities of Nazism (Silberman 2015). Confronting this history is deeply uncomfortable; health professionals want to believe that present-day society operates under a very different set of ethics. However, critically placing the medical and health professions in a historical context, as owing a debt to some of the worst moments of human history, enables us to understand some of the institutional attitudes to disability that persist today.

'Disability is not normal, not imagined, not welcomed, not needed, not common, not necessary, and not going to come to mind as the type for whom buildings are built or services provided' (Titchkosky 2008: 48). Taking healthcare as an example, NHS England only has accessibility listings for 200 of its many thousands of buildings (NHS England 2020) and disabled people report many physical barriers to accessing health services (Read et al. 2018). Yet, even if all physical barriers were removed, disabled people would still be unable to access services as freely as non-disabled people. 'Unless the relation between environment and its participants is theorized and thereby disturbed, disability will continue to be included as an excludable type, even as the physical environment changes' (Titchkosky 2008: 46).

The occupations to which access might be facilitated for disabled people fall within a spectrum that society deems acceptable for them. This is unlikely to include such activities as sex, drugs and rock'n'roll; or, to put it more formally, autotelic occupations that centre around pleasure for pleasure's sake (Csikszentmihalyi 1998). When discussing modifications to a client's home, for example, Johansson (2013) states that local authorities will often fund only 'needs' which are about 'performing activities on a basic standard level' rather than desires, which are associated with an 'excessive standard level' (p. 422). Many healthcare professionals go home to relax with a glass of wine, a cigarette or something stronger; they have sex, casual or otherwise, and enjoy themselves in any number of ways. This is understood, by them and by society at large, as a different experience from that of the patient who has been referred for 'inappropriate sexualised behaviour' or 'concerns around substance misuse' (Alexander and Gomez 2017: 117). There are risks of exploitation, abuse and health consequences for disabled people who do have sex, drink and/or drugs, just as there are for anyone; but people who require support with their activities of daily life are subjected to a high level of scrutiny about the perceived value of the activities they choose to engage in. There is very little concern with how disabled people can be supported to access the full spectrum of human experience.

Whilst the physical environment is an important aspect of access, it does not represent all of the various social and cultural practices that work together to constitute marginalisation and to grant or deny access. From a practice theory perspective, places are places for action, as discussed in Chapter 4. Places are constituted and reconstituted by the practices performed within them (Pink 2012). For example, a church building may be used at different times for a variety of social practices, such as religious services, wedding ceremonies, baptisms, choir practice and concerts. Each of these practices constitutes the building as a place for that practice: a place of worship, a place for celebration, a place for rehearsal or a place for performance. When we talk about access to a place, therefore, we are talking about access to the practice that constitutes that space at that time.

Access is not something that can be succinctly defined or taken for granted. Barriers to access are not simple oversights that can be corrected by altering a single practice; there are numerous, interwoven practices at work, from the procedural to the ideological, which knit together to produce a system where marginalised people face challenges in accessing all aspects of life. For example, Oxfam reported that the COVID-19 pandemic 'has hurt people living in poverty far harder than the rich, and has had particularly severe impacts on women, Black people, Afro-descendants, Indigenous Peoples, and historically marginalized and oppressed communities around the world' (Oxfam 2021: 14). The reason for this unequal impact is that these groups do not have the same access to healthcare, education, paid work or housing as people who are not marginalised; and the pandemic not only highlighted the gap but also increased it.

Access to everyday life

Beginning with the everyday practices that make up daily life may seem a strange choice when discussing access, which is often understood as a macro-level sociological and political phenomenon. Yet the heart of occupational therapy is the understanding that people's sense of self and ways of relating to society are produced through a 'complex dance of being, doing, becoming and belonging activities' (Clouston 2015: 36). Studying policy and high-level political decisions contributes to an understanding of barriers to access for disabled people, but it sheds little light on where and how a lack of access is most keenly felt by those who experience it:

> Fundamentally, it is necessary to theoretically grapple with questions of accessibility while not reducing access to only a political-legal issue. Every fight for access (or against it) is also an interpretive space in need of theorizing since access is always tied to the production of daily life as embodied beings.
>
> (Titchkosky 2008: 56)

Questions of access pervade every aspect of participating in a life worth living and are often enacted at the most mundane levels. Taking the ordinary experiences of everyday life as our starting point allows us to examine the multiple practices that weave together to create an oppression that is often deeply internalised in marginalised people, as it is reflected and reproduced in institutional and systematic practices that are first learned and then sustained as habitual. Indeed, it would be difficult to overestimate the extent to which barriers to access are encountered in everyday life by marginalised people (see example in Box 6.3).

Box 6.3   Barriers to access in everyday life

Participants with learning disabilities in an Australian study (Bigby et al. 2009) reflected that an activity as mundane as choosing what to have for breakfast revealed an array of social and institutional practices affecting that choice. Since one resident always chose Weetabix for breakfast, the care staff decided there was no point in buying a variety of cereals for him to choose from, as they already knew what his preference would be. This might seem like a reasonable decision on the part of care staff but the result is that someone who needs support to access the same basic rights as the rest of the population, such as freedom of choice, is restricted from doing so. His right to choice is considered less important than the time and money his residential home saves by not buying a selection of cereals.

People who are not supported to make choices pertaining to their everyday activities are unlikely to be supported with bigger choices that relate to where they live, whether or not they are given intrusive medical treatment and so on. As Kanyeredzi et al. (2019) eloquently pointed out:

> In principle, patients can do whatever they like, but they do not typically do so because the trajectories of their health and wellbeing are mapped out for them by clinical expertise in such a way that their actions are made to hang heavy with the consequences that are rendered as direct outcomes of their 'choices' (p.3).

Barriers to access in everyday life are not only encountered in institutional settings; people who have more obviously free access to come and go as they please still encounter problems (Prodinger et al. 2014). Unless barriers to access are overcome, they can contribute to **social exclusion**, which is a denial of entry to, or participation in, the prevailing social system and its rights and privileges (Oxford Languages, n.d.). For example, one woman decided to wear her own trousers into work, instead of uniform trousers, because she could not do up the button, rather than asking for uniform trousers without a button; because this would mean admitting she could not do something. She worried this would make her seem less capable and lead to losing her job.

This section has explored access as a social issue; looking at what access means, barriers to access and how these barriers create and perpetuate marginalisation and exclusion. The next section considers some of the macro-level factors that facilitate or impede access.

Macro-level access issues

When health and social care systems are viewed from a practice theory perspective, it becomes apparent that they do not exist in an apolitical, asocial, value-free vacuum. Health professionals are always acting in social practices that form within, and are shaped by, macro-systems. **Macro-systems** is an umbrella term for the culture and society that frame the structures of, and relationships among, social practices; for example, neoliberal and communist ideologies are two macro-systems that give rise to very different social structures.

A macro-system is composed of cultural patterns, values, beliefs, political structures and economic arrangements. This conceptualisation originally stems from Bronfenbrenner's (1979) Ecological Model, which was developed to explain how social environments affect children's development. The Bronfenbrenner perspective captures the complexity of the socio-cultural world; therefore, although based on an ecological approach, it provides a useful way of understanding how different system levels, from the most intimate micro-system to the most expansive macro-system, interact and have a significant influence on institutional services. Embedded in macro-systems are laws and law enforcement practices, economic systems, social and healthcare policies, political organisations etc. and their related values and symbolic forms, which together affect, shape, reinforce and change social practices. Social systems, structures and practices all work together in a dynamic interplay over time (Luhmann 2012).

Practice theory frames the concept of macro-level in a different way, with practice, not social structures, as the focal point (Schatzki 1996; Nicolini 2012). According to practice theory, practices should not be thought of as separate entities; they hang together as practice complexes and are always referred to in the plural. Blue and Spurling (2017: 27) proposed the concept of 'connective tissue' to refer to the interconnectedness of practices within complexes. In order to explain how practices both change and stay the same, they describe connective tissue as having three qualities: jurisdictional, temporal and material-spatial (Blue and Spurling 2017), as described in Box 6.4.

Box 6.4   Three qualities of connective tissue in hospital life (Blue and Spurling 2017)

Jurisdictional qualities include the ways that expert labour is divided up and allocated to different professionals; how social problems are framed by different professional groups; what tools and equipment they use; how facts are framed; professional teleology and hierarchical relationships. These divisions of responsibility affect, for instance, departmental opening hours, such as occupational therapy services only being available during the working day and clients having to fit into this. They also affect what are acknowledged as the legitimate problems on which occupational therapists are authorised to take action.

Temporal qualities refer to the socio-temporal ordering of practices, including timing, tempo, periodicity, duration, scheduling, sequencing, coordination and synchronisation. These qualities reflect the ways that practices connect across a number of temporal scales, affecting such events as referrals, hospitalisations, visiting hours, processing time and termination of treatment. For example, there may be a maximum number of treatments allocated for a particular condition or a time limit for treating a client that the occupational therapist has to conform to.

Material-spatial qualities include infrastructure, built environments, technologies and the spatial relationships between them. Schatzki (2010: 130) called these 'material arrangements', arguing that practices are both carried on amid and determinative of material arrangements. The material-spatial quality of connective tissue includes 'both the constitutive and connective features of materiality' (Blue and Spurling 2017: 32), meaning that the material elements of practice 'are both shaped by and shaping of complexes of practices'. For example, the way that hospitals are laid out is both shaped by and shapes the complex of practices that makes up hospital life. This can be seen in occupational therapy departments being located separately from wards, which places occupational therapy as an add-on service that is secondary to acute care. This placing indicates hierarchies not only of services but also of health professionals.

These three qualities define how the institution frames and delineates the task (what), the service users (who), their needs (why) and the way services are delivered (where and when). This is the mechanism that ensures occupational therapy services are reserved for pre-defined user groups and delivered in intervention formats that serve the system logic. Client groups and their needs are categorised and stereotyped to fit with institutional frames and resources. Thus, occupational therapy is not a service for everyone but only for those groups that fall within the jurisdiction of occupational therapy, as determined by the institution.

Access to occupational therapy services

When occupational therapy services are organised within institutional structures, they may not be accessible to everyone who needs them. It is the reality of occupational therapy that, within the temporal features of the institution and sites of service delivery, some people are excluded. These could be people categorised as homeless or refugees, they could be cancer survivors, or they could be people whose condition does not fit any criteria set for service by the institution (see example in Box 6.5). This situation challenges system logic (Luhmann 2012); if a change is to occur, attention needs to be paid to the macro-level logic that is enacted and visible in micro-behaviours and decisions concerning access. The jurisdiction and areas of expertise of the occupational therapist have to be negotiated, maintained and altered within the complexes of practices that make up the healthcare institution.

Box 6.5   Exclusion from occupational therapy services

Cancer survivors are a relatively new patient group that does not fit easily into treatment categories other than medical and surgical. As cancer treatment has improved, the number of cancer survivors has increased and, as a consequence, new treatment needs are emerging. Some cancer survivors have a hard time managing their everyday lives after diagnosis and treatment; they may experience side effects different from those of the acute treatment phase, and late sequelae such as pain, depression, anxiety, sexual problems and fatigue.

Awareness of these kinds of problems is increasing but realistic and effective treatment options, such as cancer rehabilitation and home-based palliative care, are not yet widely available. When treatment at the hospital is terminated, after the acute phase, care transitions to the municipality or local services. Since many countries do not have legislation mandating access for cancer survivors to occupational therapy services in the community, funding may not be available to provide occupational therapy for this client group. This is a macro-level issue of access that relates to the jurisdictional qualities of healthcare services.

Despite good intentions, high professional standards and strong values, professionals cannot avoid repeating, reproducing and reinforcing institutional policies by their actions, which are always embedded in social practices. Systems change slowly and, although errors or inadequacies may be detected, social practices are repeated (Dreier 2008). These practices have meaning for the system and are manageable within the working context, ensuring the dominance of a system-centred approach. For example, when a client is referred to occupational therapy in a hospital environment, the service may be restricted to ADL interventions, such as personal care, regardless of the client's overall life situation, personal preferences or individual needs. Service provision operates within certain structures and rationalities, as if one size fits all. When confronted with an atypical case that does not fit established protocols, the occupational therapist may feel uncertain about what to do. This creates an indissoluble tension for the therapist between system-centred and client-centred approaches.

Accessibility and availability are two distinct matters (Iwarsson and Ståhl 2003): services that society judges to be accessible to everyone may, in reality, be available only to certain groups, albeit for different reasons. For example, marginalised groups, such as ethnic minorities, may feel excluded because services are not designed to fit their cultural and linguistic expectations and needs. If a group of people is sufficiently strong, they might organise themselves as a pressure group. They may form a network and fight for access to the services from which they feel excluded. This bottom-up approach works in some cases; for example, some patient organisations for minority disability groups have succeeded in campaigning for access to occupational therapy services. This was the case in Denmark for children with sensory integration problems, who finally, after parents' campaigning, gained access to occupational therapy services in primary healthcare and not just in a hospital setting. This outcome was made possible only after changes to complexes of healthcare practices, including their jurisdictional, temporal and material-spatial features. The final and most visible change may be an amendment to the law of the country.

Examples of macro-level access issues can also be found in the ongoing digitalisation of the financial sector. Digital solutions are in general considered a good thing in the financial sector, as they increase control and have a positive impact on the safety of money, thus serving societal interests. However, as with all progressive steps, there is a downside, in that access to money may become more difficult for some citizens when services become digital, as shown in Box 6.6. For many people, financial independence is deeply connected to their sense of autonomy and managing everyday life. Sweden is one of the most digitalised countries in the world: by 2025, it is projected that half of the shops will no longer accept cash payments. This is a change that can become difficult for many consumer groups, especially the very young or the elderly. Senior citizens' groups have raised their voices against government policies for a no-cash society. They have organised public demonstrations in front of parliament buildings in a new network called 'the cash rebellion', displaying posters that proclaim 'aunts and uncles use cash'.

Box 6.6   How digital solutions can challenge the homeless

In Denmark, private banking and everyday money transactions are increasingly managed by digital solutions, to the extent that a cashless society may soon be a reality. Every citizen needs to have a bank account in order to receive social allowances or other digital income.

Recently, it has been decided that everyone must possess a credit card since bank branches are closing or performing with no cash on site, as services are centralised. To obtain a credit card, a person must have a residential address. The main characteristic of homeless people is that they have neither housing nor a residential address. So, even though credit card services are widely available in Denmark, they are not accessible to all groups. This has been described as an issue of access to money but it is also, and maybe even more importantly, an issue of access to participation in social practices that relate to handling personal finances, which is considered a basic civil right.

Not being able to handle one's personal finances, whether for structural and/ or personal reasons, is a problem of everyday living and a legitimate reason for calling upon occupational therapy services, if these services are available to homeless people without additional health problems. This example illustrates how occupational therapy services may be needed by people who do not have access to them because they belong to a group of people who are not identified as being within the jurisdiction of occupational therapy.

It is worth noting that other services may step in when occupational therapy is not available or accessible. An organisation for homeless people, called *Sand*, has negotiated a constructive, temporary solution with the banking sector that lets homeless people use the organisation's residential address as their home address in order to obtain a credit card. *Sand* also helps people, as needed, to use computers to manage their bank accounts.

Marginalised groups, in healthcare as well as in the social sector, may be deprived of occupational therapy services because they do not meet the formal criteria that bring them within the jurisdiction of those services. It may be that they are not considered to merit referral to the institutional setting or not to belong in a pre-defined client group, both of which are often tied to a specific diagnosis. In modern healthcare services, diagnosis always seems to trump needs. If the client does not have the correct diagnosis or is not in the right setting, then their need for occupational therapy is ignored due to structural issues.

As health systems are changing and healthcare is getting more specialised, the pre-defined right setting for a given treatment is increasingly being challenged, as illustrated by the following case study.

Case study 1: Ljósid – a not-for-profit cancer rehabilitation service, by Erne Magnusdóttir

In Iceland, an occupational therapist, Erna Magnusdottir, recognised that a new approach was required to meet the long-term needs of cancer patients. She responded to these needs by establishing a private–public rehabilitation service, called Ljósid, that has now been running successfully for more than 15 years (Bukhave and Creek 2021).

Ljósid offers outpatient support and rehabilitation to adults living with cancer. It came about when Magnusdóttir identified the potential of an occupation-based approach to meet the needs of cancer survivors in Iceland. Recognising that the structure of the public healthcare system could not accommodate the type of service she envisaged, she sought multi-level political and financial support, and succeeded in founding a not-for-profit organisation. The project began with private funding; at the present time, salaries for 30 members of staff are paid by the national government while additional costs are met by private funding and NGOs. Most services are free of charge, except for a nominal fee for lunch, handicraft sessions and massage therapy.

The unconventional staff group includes cosmetologists, arts and crafts tutors and health and lifestyle coaches, collaborating in an interdisciplinary team with occupational therapists, physiotherapists and psychologists. Nurses and oncologists are not part of the team but visit the centre as necessary to bring in additional expertise. This mixture of staff and funding indicates how jurisdictional qualities were challenged to create the right setting and assemble the right resources.

Magnusdóttir prioritised finding a site for Ljósid away from the hospital environment, in an area with easy access to outdoor crafting opportunities, exercise or relaxation. The location shapes how the service is perceived by service users and their relatives; creating a welcoming aura and presenting itself as a place where you want to be. In the choice of this location, the material-spatial qualities of what is considered usual for a rehabilitation centre were challenged; Magnusdóttir organised the space according to her vision of what Ljósid could be.

Since Ljósid operates as a rehabilitation service for anyone with a cancer diagnosis, referrals from doctors are not needed to get access to treatment. Service users come to the centre on their own terms; following an initial assessment, an individualised programme is developed for each person. The rehabilitation process follows individual needs so that the temporal extent can be very different, with service users attending for between three months and two years. Termination of treatment is negotiated between the service user and case manager. This exemplifies both how temporal qualities can be challenged and a truly person-centred approach. Next of kin from the age of six years also have access to the facilities and specialised resources.

Ljósid has become a great success and has changed complexes of practices related to the delivery of occupational therapy for cancer patients and survivors in Iceland. Around 100 people attend the centre every day; and about 520 per month.

This example described how an occupational therapist when she detected the emerging needs of cancer patients and survivors in her country, worked with macro-level issues to influence policymakers and financial structures. This change of practices could not have been accomplished without addressing all three qualities of the interconnectedness of practices outlined in Box 6.4. Addressing just one quality – jurisdictional, temporal or material-spatial, would not have been enough to bring about a major change.

In this section, we looked at some of the macro-level issues that influence who has access to places and practices in society and who faces barriers to access. These issues were framed as qualities of the interconnections between social practices, such as the distribution of power, the socio-temporal ordering of different practices and how space is allocated and used. We explored how some of the people who might benefit from occupational therapy services are denied access to them because they are not categorised as falling within the jurisdiction of occupational therapy.

The next section considers some of the access issues for the people who receive occupational therapy services and how the occupational therapy practitioner works with those issues.

Micro-level access issues in diverse settings

The people who might benefit from using occupational therapy services, sometimes called *patients*, *clients* or *service users*, are those experiencing difficulties with the occupations of everyday life in the contexts in which they live and work. This includes people whose occupations are limited by disability or illness and those whose opportunities are constrained by social issues, such as structural poverty, violence or displacement.

Since occupational therapists are concerned with people's everyday occupations, it would seem logical to locate occupational therapy practice in the settings where these occupations naturally take place: people's homes, communities and workplaces. However, most occupational therapy services are still located in medical and other care settings, such as hospitals and clinics, meaning that clients are expected to demonstrate and practise performance skills in simulated environments rather than in their everyday environments. Furthermore, the onus is on the client to access occupational therapy services rather than on the occupational therapist to access the client's everyday life context.

There are many ways in which occupational therapists and clients come together, either in healthcare settings or everyday life contexts. Occupational therapists who work within healthcare services often depend on referrals from other staff, such as doctors, who act as filters in deciding who would benefit from occupational therapy. In some service areas, an occupational therapist might be responsible for assessing all the patients in a particular location, such as an in-patient ward or day hospital. The filter then becomes people's eligibility for that service. When the occupational therapist works in the settings where people live and work, rather than in a healthcare setting, she is often able to identify for herself who might benefit most from occupational therapy input. For example, the occupational therapist working in a refugee camp or disaster zone can observe how people perform their everyday activities and make judgements about where, when and how to offer assistance. Furthermore, people can see what the occupational therapist is doing with others in the setting and make their own decision to join in.

We might expect it to be obvious when someone is being marginalised or excluded, but there are many reasons why we do not notice certain groups of people being left out, or even do not see them at all. The next section examines some of the social practices that create and maintain marginalisation and barriers to full access.

Barriers to access

As discussed above, some groups of people are marginalised, on the basis of differences from certain social norms, by being denied access to certain places and the social practices that are performed within them. For example, mainstream society, and the language it uses, may determine that disabled people are not deserving of access to personhood unless they conform to or mimic social norms (see example in Box 6.7). When people hide their stigmatising difference in order to access social practices that would otherwise be denied to them, this is sometimes called 'passing' (Goffman 1963/1968, p. 92).

Box 6.7   Disability and personhood

Mainstream society has historically found it difficult to accept that disabled people have the same access to personhood as non-disabled people. As autistic disability activist, Mel Baggs, poignantly reflected, through an assisted communication device:

> ... the thinking of people like me is only taken seriously if we learn your language, no matter how we previously thought or interacted ... It is only when I type something in your language that you refer to me as having communication. I smell things. I listen to things. I feel things. I taste things. I look at things. It is not enough to look and listen and taste and smell and feel, I have to do those to the right things, such as look at books, and fail to do them to the wrong things, or else people doubt that I am a thinking being. And since their definition of thought defines their definition of personhood so ridiculously much, they doubt that I am a real person as well.
>
> (SilentMiaow 2007).

Occupational therapists are not immune to the social forces at play and to the conceptualisation of disabled people in popular consciousness that these social forces create. Curran (2016: 435) suggested that incidents of ableism from healthcare professionals are not 'examples of "poor practice" or types of individual but the effects of continuous normalising strategies that contribute to wider societal discourses'. When occupational therapists are influenced by social norms and, in turn, reinscribe marginalising ways of conceptualising disabled people, they can reinforce barriers to access.

People may be denied access to certain social practices because those practices are considered too risky to the individual, to others or to social structures. **Risk** is the possibility of danger (Lupton 1999); high risk means a strong likelihood of the danger occurring, while low risk means a slight possibility. For example, a person with a mental illness diagnosis may be detained in hospital against his will because he is seen as having a high suicide risk. A prisoner may be denied parole and release into the community because she is thought to be a risk to society. During the COVID-19 pandemic, people in many countries were not allowed to meet in large social groups because of the perceived risks of spreading the disease and overwhelming health services.

Some situations pose a real and immediate risk, which must be managed. However, the organisational response, when questions of access, rights and dignity are proposed, tends to be that safety comes first. It may be argued that ensuring people's physical safety is crucial to enabling access, but considerations of risk are only part of the picture. For example, managing the risk of personal injury was historically viewed as a key criterion for assessing whether a psychiatric in-patient was fit to be released from their detention (Stein 2002). But people with certain mental illness diagnoses, such as borderline personality disorder, may always engage in some degree of self-harm in response to overwhelming emotional trauma (Brodsky and Stanley 2013). Focusing solely on risks may mean that scant attention is paid to how people who self-harm are granted or denied access to everyday life (James et al. 2017).

We will now think about some of the approaches used by occupational therapists to address access issues.

Enabling access

As described above, occupational therapists have the expertise to facilitate access for many different groups of people, not just those experiencing illness or disability. Having access to a range of occupations, and the social practices of which they form a part, can be seen as an issue of social justice. Many health and social care problems come, directly or indirectly, from people being excluded from mainstream society; therefore, solutions to these problems lie not in the individual or their immediate environment but in social systems. There is a pressing need for occupational therapists to question the value of using their time to patch up a broken health and social care system, fixing single issues for individuals while knowing that the same issue will recur again and again. Instead, the profession could pay more attention to challenging those systems that do not work for whole sections of the population around the world.

In order to assist people experiencing access problems, the occupational therapist has to be able to recognise what the issues are and frame them in ways that suggest appropriate responses (Creek and Cook 2017). An example of this is given in Box 6.8.

Box 6.8   Naming and framing an access problem

An occupational therapist, Sue, worked with a charity providing outdoor activity respite for UK army veterans. The older veterans had served in Northern Ireland, during the conflict of the second half of the 20th century, while younger veterans had been in Afghanistan or Iraq. Most of them were currently unemployed and many were experiencing problems with drugs, alcohol, depression and physical health problems. One way of understanding their situation would be to frame it as post-traumatic stress disorder (PTSD).

Sue noted that men had often chosen to join the army because there was a shortage of other jobs in the areas where they lived. Joining the army gave them access to many benefits: paid work; companionship; purpose; structure in their daily lives; a social role and a positive sense of identity. On leaving the army, they lost most of these benefits, often finding themselves returning to live in areas of social and economic deprivation and encountering additional difficulty adapting to civilian life. During the activity holiday, participants found themselves once more belonging to a community, working with other ex-soldiers and recreating an occupational and cultural identity.

Sue formulated the veterans' problems in terms of loss of connection; connection with other people, with valued occupations and with a culture they felt part of. She observed that the connections made during the activity break could not be sustained when participants went home: new connections had been established just to be lost again. Sue noted that this could be harmful rather than beneficial for participants' mental and physical health.

This formulation of the health difficulties of army veterans, as loss of connection to valued relationships and occupations, led Sue to understand that the veterans needed follow-up occupational therapy services at home to help them access new occupations and build healthy, lasting connections in their local neighbourhoods and communities.

Some occupational therapists are finding new ways to address systemic issues, such as endemic poverty and structural discrimination. In Brazil, for example, social occupational therapy is prompting practitioners to work alongside their clients to demand systemic change. Heavily influenced by radical educator, Paulo Freire (1972), social occupational therapy builds on the notion that, just as students should not be treated as empty vessels to be filled with knowledge by an omniscient teacher, so those who use occupational therapy services should not be seen as broken people who can only be fixed with the expert knowledge that professionals provide. Understanding people as co-creators of knowledge and experts by experience allows occupational therapists to collaboratively identify systemic barriers to access and fight alongside their clients to remove these barriers for everyone.

Enabling access is about achieving equity rather than promoting equality. **Equality** means giving each individual or group of people the same quantity of resources or opportunities; **equity** is justice or fairness (Shorter Oxford English Dictionary 2002). The concept of equity carries the implication that each person has different circumstances and would need to be allocated particular resources and opportunities in order to reach an equal outcome. For example, a ramp may be necessary for wheelchair users to be able to access a building that has steps at all entrances.

Case study 2 describes the work of an occupational therapist in the UK, whose job is to facilitate access to higher education for students with disabilities.

Case study 2: Specialist mentoring for university students, by Lesley McCallion

Anne is an occupational therapist with 37 years of clinical experience, together with additional training in body psychotherapy. Anne works part-time in a new area of practice, as a specialist mentor for mental health with university students; a role she has now held for two-and-a-half years.

The students who see Anne are of varying ages, from 18 upwards. Their assessed disability, in the context of the disabled student allowance (DSA) for which they are eligible, is either: (1) specific learning-related difficulty, including different ways of learning and of relating to others and to the environment, due to neurodivergent patterns such as dyslexia or ADHD, or (2) mental health condition, such as depression or anxiety (GOV.UK 2021).

The role of specialist mentor requires that the post-holder be a registered healthcare professional and that they have relevant work experience. It is made clear that they are not employed to work as a psychotherapist or counsellor; rather, the role is to use their specialist knowledge to support students in managing the demands of academic life, including the social and personal aspects of being a student.

All students are seen individually by their specialist mentors, many of them online. The number of hours is allocated on the basis of the DSA assessment and on medical and other evidence provided by the student in support of their application. It is the mentor's responsibility to manage the overall regulation of meetings so that a student's allocation of hours is appropriately spaced throughout the academic year.

In broad terms, Anne's role is to facilitate students' access to the university courses they have chosen, by working with them to develop effective strategies for managing their disabilities. Being a specialist mentor entails a different way of working from any that Anne had experienced previously and she has had to learn on the job how best to fulfil her role. Rather than offering a prescriptive approach, that uses pre-determined assessments, interventions and tools with each client, Anne works instead with principles, parameters and intentions. Through creating a reliable and consistent structure, she hopes to foster a way for the client to come to meetings and feel free to express their strengths, needs, goals and wishes in their own way, together with exploring with Anne the selected occupations through which they will gradually realise their own goals (see example in Box 6.9).

Box 6.9   Working with the client

A student identified feeling isolated and depressed at university. They felt this was a similar situation to one experienced earlier, at college, and they wanted to be able to interact to their own satisfaction with peers to improve their social life, enhance their mental well-being and, in turn, support their ability to study. They stated that the only time they were able to practise social interactions in a safe enough environment was during some parts of meetings with the specialist mentor.

   The student built confidence in two ways: first, by engaging with the mentor in practising how to initiate and manage conversations; and, second, by receiving feedback and support about their strengths and needs in the activity, then using it when trying to engage with others at student society events. The student had high levels of funding to support their assessed neurodivergence, which meant that meetings with the mentor could be extended beyond semester dates.

Principles offer a foundation of beliefs and propositions from which intentions can be derived. An **intention** can be defined as both a plan and a direction. Anne also defines an intention as a deliberate approach to be used that involves many factors, including, amongst others: her preparation; attention to her own state of nervous arousal and its potential impact on the client; the environmental surroundings she selects, including objects, colours and her personal appearance; her inner demeanour and thoughts about her work and her client, as well as her external presentation in terms of body language, verbal language, tone, pace and timbre. All these factors are important in face-to-face meetings but become even more significant when working online with clients.

In order for Anne to act according to principles and intentions, she develops **parameters** with each client, to provide a structure that acknowledges boundaries of time, confidentiality, privacy and appropriateness. There is an agenda, or statement of purpose, for each meeting or set of meetings but Anne does not find it helpful to have a list of points to cover or a menu of interventions. She works in the moment, rather than building up a series of questions that may never unravel the heart of the matter with the individual concerned. This way of working calls for Anne to make rapid assessments and to adapt her approach, based on the emergent dynamic between her and the student.

Anne considers a number of axes when working with clients. One such axis is time. At the simplest level, Anne takes responsibility for the length of time the meeting will last. At another level, working with nothing but the screen and image, and the visible areas behind the client and herself, it is important for her to consider time as a therapeutic tool so that past experiences and perception of self can be worked with in order to amplify recognition of current dilemmas and difficulties the client wishes to resolve. Recognising and acknowledging patterns of behaviour and experience that either have or have not served the client allows them to see whether their approach could be altered. Clients often see for themselves how to make changes but, if they do not, Anne can make suggestions for them to consider (see example in Box 6.10).

Box 6.10   Basing practice on principles

A client explains to Anne they are becoming low in mood and anxious because they are unable to turn up to lectures on time or manage deadlines for workloads, due to a perceived lack of skill in time management. Anne gently challenges this perception, on the basis that over a period of time the client turns up regularly for their meetings with her, without any prompting. In discussing how the client manages their home life and travel, it emerges that they also successfully and regularly negotiate complex train and bus timetables and the requirements of their children's schooling timetables.

Anne uses activity analysis to break down and compare the successfully and unsuccessfully managed activities and to identify both the parallel and disparate skills required. This understanding informs the activity challenge she decides to present to the client. She states her findings in practical and non-shaming language, exactly as they appear to be, in such a way that the client is able to assimilate and process the information. This allows them the opportunity to see patterns of behaviour not previously recognised.

Later, Anne works with the same client to help them recognise their alertness and pleasure in undertaking differing activities, through a comparison of the client's valued hobby, crochet, with a non-valued activity, knitting. With support from Anne, the client becomes aware of both the subtle and more obvious differences in cognitive awareness, mood and bodily sensation between the two activities. Anne then harnesses this awareness to amplify the client's ability to recognise which challenges are genuinely interesting, stimulating and pleasurable to them and which are not. Anne is careful not to imply or make any value judgement about the client's selected activities; they are free to make their own choices.

Eventually, the client realised that their perceived lack of competence was, in reality, the dissonance aroused by doing a degree they were not genuinely interested in (accountancy). Subsequently, they successfully switched to a different degree programme that favoured their passion for history.

Exploring an individual's balance of activity between work, leisure, sleep and self care provides Anne and her client with a baseline for ongoing assessment, where the client's experience of themselves, their mood and their activities can be explored. Each client's pattern of activity is unique to them; for example, Anne knows that the occupation of yoga might be physical and spiritual self-care for one person and leisure for another. The focus on everyday activity ensures that the approach is relevant to the client and they quickly learn to use it in building their sense of self-efficacy and their own expertise in healthy ways. For example, a student who sometimes misses their bus to lectures chooses to practise assertiveness techniques through role-play, to enable them to build confidence to enter the lecture late rather than avoiding going in at all.

Another aspect of the client's patterns and balance of activity is how easy or difficult they find it to bring their own intentions into action. When forming her overall impression of a client, Anne thinks in terms of 'horizontal' and 'vertical' axes; that is, a focus on the present and a future perspective. She and the client may move between these two axes within a single meeting or over the course of the relationship, according to need, as illustrated in Box 6.11.

Box 6.11   Temporal considerations

For some time, Anne has been working with a student who has severe fibromyalgia, helping them to identify that they frequently misjudge how much activity they can manage to do in a day. Their unmet expectations frequently leave them depressed, dissatisfied and unable to cope.

Taking a 'horizontal' approach, Anne works with the student to help them adjust their goals. In discussion, it emerges that, in younger years, the student was often shamed for laziness and lack of effort, both at school and at home. During their meetings, Anne encourages the student to go at a slow but adequate pace and encourages them to end the meeting when they realise they are tired. Anne is careful not to suggest that there is any judgement of the client's capabilities; even her vocal tones are very gentle. By her own way of performing, Anne encourages the student not to overstep the healthy boundaries they are learning to set in order to better manage their academic role in the long run. The message Anne gives is, 'I believe in you. You can do this if you believe in yourself and your body's need to recover and build stamina, incrementally in your own time, and if you work at a pace that is right for you whilst fulfilling your academic role'.

Later in the work with the same student, Anne encourages a more 'vertical axis', where the student lists the things they want to go out and get in the future: a big, powerful car, a suit and a salary. Anne works playfully with the client, encouraging them to have fun envisaging the size of the car and salary. This strategy helps the student not to feel they just have to work studiously until buying a Bugatti becomes a reality.

There is a lot for Anne to bear in mind during sessions, whilst also focussing on the client. Anne's approach is based on a structure designed to give freedom of expression to the client without controlling or directing what happens in meetings. Within this structure, Anne can be receptive to material that is incipient or latent in the client, using this to promote growth and change.

Summary and conclusion

This chapter has explored an issue at the heart of occupational therapy practice; access. It began by defining access in the context of occupational therapy and justifying why it is important for the profession to acknowledge and address. We then identified some of the multiple barriers to access that are produced by a complex narrative of practices, at both macro and micro-levels of society, arguing that occupational therapists have a key role to play in facilitating greater access to all areas of life. We attempted to show how problems of access are deeply woven into the fabric of society, so that bringing about change can seem like an overwhelming, if not impossible, task for the therapist.

We argued that occupational therapists are well-placed to fight barriers to access at both macro and micro-levels of society; that is, to critique the systems within which we work as well as supporting individuals and groups in overcoming barriers. The strength of the profession is in our focus on assessing physical and social environments while, at the same time, acknowledging that the challenges faced by individuals are likely to be located, at least in part, somewhere outside their own locus of control.

The next chapter covers another key topic for occupational therapists: resources.

References

Alexander, N., and Gomez, M.T. (2017) Pleasure, sex, prohibition, intellectual disability and dangerous ideas. *Reproductive Health Matters*, 25(50): 114–120. https://doi.org/10.1080/09688080.2017.1331690

Baggs, M. (2007) In my language. Online at https://www.youtube.com/watch?v=JnylM1hI2jc. Accessed May 2022.

Barnes, C., Mercer, T., and Shakespeare, T. (2010) The social model of disability. In: A. Giddens and P.W. Sutton (eds) *Sociology: introductory readings, 3rd edition*. Cambridge: Polity Press.

Bigby, C., Clement, T., Mansell, J., and Beadle-Brown, J. (2009) 'It's pretty hard with our ones, they can't talk, the more able bodied can participate': staff attitudes about the applicability of disability policies to people with severe and profound intellectual disabilities. *Journal of Intellectual Disability Research*, 53(4): 363–376.

Blue, S., and Spurling, N. (2017) Qualities of connective tissue in hospital life. In: A. Hui, T. Schatzki and E. Shove (eds.) *The nexus of practices*. Abingdon: Routledge. 24–37.

Brodsky, B., and Stanley, B. (2013) *The dialectical behavior therapy primer: how DBT can inform clinical practice*. Chichester: John Wiley and Sons.

Bronfenbrenner, U. (1979) *The ecology of human development: experiments by nature and design*. Cambridge, MA: Harvard University Press.

Bukhave, E., and Creek, J. (2021) Kreative aktiviteter som en vej til glæde og livskvalitet. [Creative activities as a way to happiness and quality of life]. In: L. Lindahl-Jacobsen and D.V. Poulsen (eds.) *Ergoterapi og fysioterapi I den palliative praksis*. København: Gad.

Changing Places (2020) Online http://www.changing-places.org/. Accessed May 2022.

Clouston, T.J. (2015) *Challenging stress, burnout and rust-out: finding balance in busy lives*. London: Jessica Kingsley Publishers.

Creek, J., and Cook, S. (2017) Learning from the margins: Enabling effective occupational therapy. *Journal of Occupational Therapy*, 80(7): 423–431.

Csikszentmihalyi, M. (1998) *Finding flow: the psychology of engagement with everyday life*. New York: Basic Books.

Curran, T. (2016) Book Review: Foucault and the government of disability. *Disability and Society*, 31(3): 434–437.

Dreier, O. (2008) *Psychotherapy in everyday life*. Cambridge: Cambridge University Press.

Duncan, M., and Creek, J. (2014) Working on the margins: occupational therapy and social inclusion. In: W. Bryant, J. Fieldhouse and K. Banningan (eds.) *Creek's occupational therapy and mental health*, 5th ed. Edinburgh: Churchill Livingstone Elsevier. 457–473.

Form, W., and Wilterdink, N. (n.d.) "Social structure". Encyclopedia Britannica. Online at https://www.britannica.com/topic/social-structure. Accessed August 2021.

Freire, P. (1972) *Pedagogy of the oppressed*. Trans. M.B. Ramos. London: Penguin.

Goffman, E. (1963/1968) *Stigma: notes on the management of spoiled identity*. Harmondsworth: Pelican.

Iwarssson, S., and Ståhl, A. (2003) Accessibility, usability and universal design–positioning and definition of concepts describing person-environment relationships. *Disability and Rehabilitation*, 25(2): 57–66.

James, K., Samuels, I., Moran, P., and Stewart, D. (2017) Harm reduction as a strategy for supporting people who self-harm on mental health wards: the views and experiences of practitioners. *Journal of Affective Disorders*, 214: 67–73.

Jamrozik, A., Oraa Ali, M., Sarwer, D., and Chatterjee, A. (2019) More than skin deep: judgments of individuals with facial disfigurement. *Psychology of Aesthetics, Creativity, and the Arts*, 13: 117–129. 10.1037/aca0000147

Johansson, K. (2013) Have they done what they should? Moral reasoning in the context of translating older person's everyday problems into eligible needs for home modification services. *Medical Anthropology Quarterly*, 27(3): 414–433.

Kanyeredzi, A., Brown, S., McGrath, L., Reavey, P., and Tucker, I. (2019) The atmosphere of the ward: attunements and attachments of everyday life for patients on a medium-secure forensic psychiatric unit. *The Sociological Review Monographs*, 67 (2): 444–466.

Luhmann, N. (2012) *Introduction to systems theory*. Chichester: Wiley.

Lupton, D. (1999) *Risk*. London: Routledge.

MENCAP (2012) Death by indifference: 74 deaths and counting. A progress report 5 years on. Online at https://www.mencap.org.uk/sites/default/files/2016-08/Death%20by%20Indifference%20-%2074%20deaths%20and%20counting.pdf. Accessed: May 2022.

MENCAP (2018). Treat me well: simple adjustments make a big difference. Online at https://www.mencap.org.uk/sites/default/files/2018-07/2017.005.01%20Campaign%20report%20digital.pdf. Accessed May 2022.

Morton-Nance, S., and Schafer, T. (2012) End of life care for people with a learning disability. *Nursing Standard*, 27(1): 40–47.

Mosey, A.C. (1986) *Psychosocial components of occupational therapy*. New York: Raven Press.

Natasha, A., and Gomez, M.T. (2017) Pleasure, sex, prohibition, intellectual disability, and dangerous ideas. *Reproductive Health Matters*, 25(50): 114–120.

NHS England (2020) Accessing NHS buildings. Online at https://www.property.nhs.uk/property/accessable/. Accessed May 2022.

Nicolini, D. (2012) *Practice theory, work and organization*. Oxford: Oxford University Press.

Oxfam (2021) *The inequality virus*. Oxford: Oxfam International.

Oxford Languages (n.d.) English dictionary. Online at https://languages.oup.com/google-dictionary-en/. Accessed May 2022.

Pink, S. (2012) *Situating everyday life*. Los Angeles: Sage.

Prodinger, B., Shaw, L., Laliberte Rudman, D., and Stamm, T. (2014) Negotiating disability in everyday life: ethnographical accounts of women with rheumatoid arthritis. *Disability and Rehabilitation*, 36(6): 497–503.

Read, S., Heslop, P., Turner, S., Mason-Angelow, V., Tilbury, N., Miles, C., and Hatton, C. (2018). Disabled people's experiences of accessing reasonable adjustments in hospitals: a qualitative study. *BMC Health Services Research*, 18(1): 931. 10.1186/s12913-018-3757-7

Regnard, C., Matthews, D., Gibson, L., and Clarke, C. (2003) Difficulties in identifying distress and its causes in people with severe communication problems. *International Journal of Palliative Nursing*, 9: 173–176.

Sawyer, A., and Bright, K. (2014) *The access manual: auditing and managing inclusive built environments*. Chichester: Wiley-Blackwell.

Schatzki, T.R. (1996) *Social practices: a Wittgensteinian approach to human activity and the social*. Cambridge: Cambridge University Press.

Schatzki, T. (2010) Materiality and social life. *Nature and Culture*, 5(2): 123–149.

Shorter Oxford English Dictionary (2002) Oxford: Oxford University Press.

Silberman, S. (2015) *NeuroTribes: the legacy of autism and the future of neurodiversity.* New York: Avery.

SilentMiaow (2007) In my language. Online at https://www.youtube.com/watch?v= JnylM1hI2jc. Accessed May 2022.

Stein, W. (2002) The use of discharge risk assessment tools in general psychiatric services in the UK. *Journal of Psychiatric and Mental Health Nursing,* 9: 713–724.

Stephenson, J. (2018) Fresh warnings over future of learning disability nursing raised at summit meeting. Online at https://www.nursingtimes.net/news/education/fresh-warnings-raised-on-future-of-learning-disability-nursing/7025485.article. Accessed May 2022.

Stone, A., and Wright, T. (2013) When your face doesn't fit: employment discrimination against people with facial disfigurements. *Journal of Applied Social Psychology,* 43: 515–526.

Thornton, J. (2019) People with learning disabilities have lower life expectancy and cancer screening rates. *British Medical Journal,* 364: 1404.

Titchkosky, T. (2008) "To pee or not to pee?" Ordinary talk about extraordinary exclusions in a university environment. *Canadian Journal of Sociology/Cahiers Canadiens de Sociologie,* 33(1): 37–60.

Trade Union Congress (2017) Mental Health and Employment. Online at https://www.tuc.org.uk/sites/default/files/Mental_Health_and_Employment.pdf. Accessed May 2022.

Welch, M. (1990) Disabled climb capitol steps to plead for government protection. Online at https://apnews.com/2672c50ca9c6155ed0cc3a4e36bdc20c05/08/2020

Whybrow, S., and Bridge, C. (2015) Accessibility outcomes in disaster recovery – a critical concern, a minimum requirement or an afterthought? In: N. Rushford and K. Thomas (eds.) *Disaster and development: an occupational perspective.* Edinburgh: Elsevier/WFOT. 129–137.

7 Resources

Temple Moore and Jennifer Creek

Introduction

Chapter 6 discussed issues around gaining access to the groups that would be likely to benefit most from occupational therapy intervention in diverse settings. This chapter explores issues around resourcing occupational therapy practice in diverse settings.

Many of the work settings described in this book, such as refugee camps and community centres, either lack resources found in traditional occupational therapy settings or have different material and human resources than those typically encountered. This affects the occupations of people living in or otherwise occupying the setting and of occupational therapists working there. For example, homeless people staying in emergency overnight accommodation will not have access to all the resources available in long-term housing. Equally, the occupational therapist working in this setting will not have access to the equipment, space and expertise found in a hospital or clinic setting.

The chapter begins with an explanation of the people and things that constitute resources for occupational therapy practice: personal capabilities, material resources, space-time and human resources. It then considers how macro-level factors, including economics and politics, influence resource availability and use in diverse settings. This is followed by an exploration of micro-level resource issues, illustrated with a real-life case study of occupational therapy practice in a marginal setting. The chapter finishes with a brief section on resourcefulness as a professional competence, illustrated with a second case study.

What are resources?

When an occupational therapist thinks about what people do, this always includes consideration of the physical and social spaces where performance takes place. As discussed in Chapter 4, a space is a place where practices are performed: '... space is itself defined by what goes on within it' (Shove, Pantzar and Watson 2012: 132). Occupational performance is understood to occur in both objective, physical spaces and relational, social spaces. Take a church, for example, there is a church building, where services and other meetings take place at specified times; this is the objective, physical space of the church. There are also clergy, congregation, choir and caretakers, who have their own roles and relationships within the church community; these form the relational, social space of the church. In analysing a person's occupations, the

DOI: 10.4324/9781003016755-7

Table 7.1 Resources for occupational therapy

Personal capabilities	Material resources	Space-time	Human resources
Competences	Objects	Setting	Time
Meanings	Artefacts	Doing-place	Energy
Motivations	Technologies and infrastructures	History	Competences
	Tools and hardware	Future orientation	Knowledge

therapist takes note of the human and non-human resources that form part of spaces, as they influence, support or inhibit occupational performance.

A **resource** is a stock or reserve that can be drawn on as needed (Shorter Oxford English Dictionary 2002). Resources that can be drawn on for occupational performance include personal capabilities, materials, space-time and other people, as shown in Table 7.1.

In Chapter 1, occupations as social practices were defined as 'routine, bodily activities made possible by the active contribution of an array of material resources' (Nicolini 2012: 4). This definition includes materials as necessary, constitutive components of occupational performance: there can be no performance without bodies and other material resources. The body itself has been described as a material resource, together with objects, consumer goods (Blue et al. 2014), artefacts, technologies, tools and hardware (Shove, Pantzar and Watson 2012).

Occupations are embodied; therefore, the body, with its mental and physical competences, is a necessary resource for occupational performance. **Competences** are 'the personal preconditions that enable a person to participate in a social practice' (Dreier 2008: 33). They include know-how, practical skills and tacit understanding. Personal competences are developed through activity in the world and a person only has competences in relation to the possibilities afforded by particular contexts, together with the material resources they contain (Dreier 2008).

Material resources are objects in the environment that form necessary components of many occupations. Owing to the dependence of many performances on material resources, occupations can be described as routinised relations between people and objects (Reckwitz 2002). For example, a ball and goals, or improvised alternatives, are indispensable resources for playing football; without these materials, players would not be able to agree on the rules of how the game will be played.

All occupational performance takes place in space and time, which are themselves mutually constitutive: space does not exist without time and time does not exist without space (see Chapter 3). The concept of **space-time** makes the point that everything people do has a setting and a history, that occupational performances integrate past and future and that time and space are united in the moment of performance (Shove, Pantzar and Watson 2012). This means that a social practice does not just exist in the here and now but is always the product of tradition and custom, through which the purpose and meaning of the practice have evolved. Awareness of the personal, social and cultural meanings of occupations might be especially significant in working with marginal communities, and those where cultural integrity or identity is fragile.

Hui and Walker (2018) used the term **doing-places** to refer to the spaces within which the performance of particular types of activity is possible. For example, a kitchen might be a doing-place for cooking; as well as for other activities, such as washing up, making coffee and cleaning. When we talk about space, we often mean physical space, such as a football pitch, but spaces can also be virtual. We occupy physical and virtual spaces at the same time. For example, when two people in different places are having a conversation online, they each occupy a separate physical space while simultaneously sharing the virtual space of the online interaction. People living in different parts of the world may operate in different time zones, necessitating the negotiation of an agreed time to meet online. The time is the same for both of them in the virtual space of the meeting but different in the physical spaces from which they are speaking.

A fourth resource for occupational performance is **human resources**; some occupations, such as football, depend on the participation of more than one person for their performance. People can be seen as resources in that they bring their capabilities, knowledge, time and energy to shared performances. Occupational therapists, for example, can be described as human resources for people who need help and support with their occupational lives. Even when not physically present during a performance, human resources may have been involved in providing the necessary material resources and space-time for the occupation to be performed. For example, many people will have been involved in growing, processing and distributing the ingredients used in cooking a meal.

Personal capabilities, material resources, space-time and other people make up the field of possibilities for action in any particular situation. In this sense, they can be described as affordances. An **affordance** is a relationship between the capabilities of the performer and the properties of resources in the environment, particularly material resources, that pre-figures how those resources might be used (Norman 2013). An object becomes a potential resource when the performer is able to see how it might be used and has the capabilities to use it: for example, when a dog's lead breaks while it is being walked, the owner might improvise a temporary one from his own leather belt. **Constraints** are delimitations of the field of possibilities that exclude certain courses of action and leave others open. Constraints might be due to a lack of material objects in the environment, such as there being nothing immediately available that could potentially be used as a dog lead, or to the dog walker not having the capability to see the possibility of using something else as a temporary lead.

Macro-level resource issues in diverse settings

Occupational performance depends on the availability of resources: 'What people can positively achieve is influenced by economic opportunities, political liberties, social powers and the enabling conditions of good health, basic education, and the encouragement and cultivation of initiatives' (Sen 1999: 5). In other words, access to resources in any particular local context is influenced by numerous, large-scale political and economic practices that may be distant from that context in time and space. Very large projects, including those that operate across national boundaries, are likely to require extensive negotiation and co-operation between many powerful groups and organisations (see example in Box 7.1).

Box 7.1 Negotiating resource allocation at the macro-level

The decision to build the Three Gorges dam in China, designed to protect the lives and livelihoods of people from flooding of the Yangtze River, was a huge project based on political, economic, technological and social considerations. The project only began after many years of discussion, planning and negotiation. However, concern for the well-being of local people was only one factor in the decision to build the dam, which also served the economic interests of the Chinese government and big business.

The local benefits of major infrastructure projects can be highly debatable, especially when set against the negative consequences for local communities, such as the devaluing or destruction of homes, fractured and stagnating communities and generations affected by worry and displacement.

Economic opportunities, political liberties and social powers are important, large-scale influences on resource availability. **Economics** refers to practices associated with the production and distribution of wealth within a state. **Politics** refers to the practices involved in governing, organising and administering a state. In a globalised world, many economic and political influences extend across state boundaries. For the purposes of this chapter, **power** has two meanings: 'the capacity to act with effect', which is the power of individuals; and 'the capacity to direct or purposively influence the actions of others' (Watson 2017: 170), which is exercised on a large scale through political and economic practices, such as policy making, mandating, trading and funding.

Decisions and actions taken at the level of the state shape the availability of resources at all levels of society, including what there is in the environment; the conditions under which potential resources can be accessed, and who has the capabilities to use the available resources. 'Social patterns such as the division of labour, gender relations, and unequal access to resources, as well as political, economic, legal, and cultural institutions are constituted by practices, but they also provide a context for the performance of practices' (Røpke 2009: 2493). Within communities, resources are not distributed equally or according to need but are allocated and accumulated in ways that tend to reproduce themselves, leading to systematised inequality that increases over time.

This section considers how economic and political influences affect the availability of personal capabilities, material resources, space-time and human resources for occupational therapy practice.

Personal capabilities: Macro-level issues

Personal capabilities are 'those things which constitute the capacity to act' (Watson 2017: 173), including know-how, practical skills, tacit understanding and dispositions (Schatzki 2001). Personal capabilities are necessary for effective utilisation of and interaction with resources in the environment. The Nobel Prize-winning economist, Amartya Sen (1999), argued that having access to material resources does not lead to flourishing unless a person also has the relevant competences for using those resources to promote her or his valued ends.

As described above, personal capabilities develop through activity in the world (Dreier 2008) and people who lack opportunities for engaging in activity, for whatever reason, do not develop the same range of competences as those who have many and varied opportunities. In this way, inequality of access to societal resources, such as good nutrition, housing, clean water, education and healthcare, results in some groups having less well-developed competences than others. 'These differences, and the processes through which they come about and are maintained, constitute the grounds of systematic social differences' (Watson 2017: 173). An example of this is given in Box 7.2.

Box 7.2   Unequal opportunities for development

Being able to read is a key competence that enables someone to take advantage of a range of opportunities, access information, communicate and understand printed instructions, including road signs and timetables. Reading proficiency is strongly associated with higher hourly wages (OECD 2013). People who cannot read are therefore disadvantaged in society, and this disadvantage is not distributed equally across countries and communities. According to UNICEF (2019), illiteracy is highest in the least developed countries and higher among females than males. Within developed countries, people from lower socio-economic backgrounds have lower rates of literacy and the educational level of parents is associated with proficiency in literacy in their children.

Material resources: Macro-level issues

Objects, consumer goods, artefacts, technologies, tools and hardware have the potential to become material resources for the performance of activities and occupations. Shove (2017) pointed out that these material resources play different roles in the performance of activities, roles that she called infrastructures, devices and resources.

Infrastructures are things that are necessary for performance 'but are not engaged with directly' (Shove 2017: 156). Examples of infrastructures include the arrangements through which electricity, data and water are distributed to communities; rail and road networks; airports, and public buildings, such as schools. **Devices** are things that are directly used in the performance of activities and occupations, such as tools, appliances and utensils (Shove 2017). Shove used the term **resources** to refer to things that are used up or transformed during the performance: occupational therapists would be more likely to call them **consumables**. Consumable resources include energy, packaging, ingredients, food and water. An example of how material resources play the roles of infrastructure, devices and consumables is given in Box 7.3.

Box 7.3 Infrastructure, devices and consumables in the kitchen

A typical kitchen in a middle-income household contains numerous devices that are used in the preparation of meals, such as bowls, pans, ovens, fridges and kettles. Some of these devices are dependent upon specific consumable resources to enable their use; for example, electric kettles require electricity. These consumables reach the kitchen via national infrastructures that provide and distribute electricity, gas and water. Other consumables, such as vegetables, cooking oil and meat, are bought and stored in the kitchen until they are used.

Access to infrastructures, devices and consumables is influenced by the same, large-scale political and economic practices that determine the availability and distribution of other types of resources. Some consumable resources can be supplied by infrastructures, including water, electricity and information. However, a developing country is likely to have less extensive national infrastructures than a developed one, in terms of extent, quality and reliability, with the consequences mainly affecting poorer people. For example, if access to a water supply and electricity is restricted by lack of infrastructure, then food preparation and bathing will be more complex while washing and drying clothes will involve extensive manual labour. Carrying water occupies a lot of time in all these tasks. Even in developed countries, infrastructures may not extend to all sectors of the population. The building and maintenance of infrastructural arrangements, such as roads and reservoirs, is strongly influenced by government policy, which is in turn shaped by the interests of different, powerful groups.

Where comprehensive infrastructures are not available, consumable resources are often acquired through manual labour, such as grinding grain by hand, carrying water from wells and collecting fuel for cooking fires. Some devices require manual labour for their use, such as a hand pump. Other devices can only be used in conjunction with particular infrastructural arrangements; for example, electric cars cannot be used without roads and a network of charging points.

People who have access to effective infrastructures and devices may need to expend less effort in acquiring consumables than people who lack such access. However, in well-resourced communities, there may be pressure for people to acquire more and more consumer goods, such as food processors, microwave ovens and bread-making machines, beyond the point of their usefulness in everyday life, just to keep up with the neighbours. Parents may find themselves working long hours to provide their children with luxury electronic goods that they have been encouraged to see as necessary.

Space-time: Macro-level issues

Every performance of activities and occupations depends on the coming together and integration of human and non-human resources in space and time. This coming together of resources depends on macro-level arrangements, such as transport infrastructures and universally agreed time zones. The spatial organisation and timing of any performance involve having the necessary resources available and accessible, including space for storing unused resources, space for the performance of activities and time for activities to be performed. Human and non-human resources may be separate in space and time until they come together during the performance (Shove 2017); an example of this is given in Box 7.4.

Box 7.4   Training for staff working with child refugees

A UK-based charity identified that staff working in child-friendly spaces in three refugee camps in Northern Uganda found it difficult to engage some of the children in their activities. The charity sponsored a small team from the United Kingdom to travel to Uganda and deliver a five-day training programme to 12 staff members working in the child-friendly spaces. The human resources for this project included: staff at the refugee camps; the three trainers; administrators and managers of refugee services in Uganda and in the United Kingdom, and children who would take part in the training programme. All these people had to be identified, recruited and brought together in space and time for the programme. Some resources for the project, such as laptop computers, were not readily available in Northern Uganda and were sent to the camps before the trainers arrived.

There are various ways in which large-scale economic, political and social factors influence how much space and time people are able to claim for performing their occupations and activities. Poor or marginalised people are less likely to own or have access to physical doing-places and spaces, such as houses, gardens and workplaces, so they depend on others to provide these facilities. This makes them vulnerable to losing their places in the world if they cannot afford to pay rent, or if the landlord decides to change how his property is used. Low-cost rental properties are likely to be located in deprived areas so that tenants may not have easy access to open public spaces, such as parks and gardens. In some countries, governments legislate to grant rights to people who rent a property or provide low-cost public housing for rent, but not all governments see this as part of their role.

Some countries set a minimum rate of pay for workers, although this may be resisted by powerful groups, such as manufacturers. The provision of state benefits to support the low paid makes it possible for employers to maintain low wages (Abramsky 2013). Many people with low incomes work long hours for a low hourly rate, often in poor working conditions, leaving little time or energy for other activities. In very poor families, children may have to work to supplement the family income, instead of going to school: the immediate economic needs of the family prevail over the possible long-term benefits of gaining an education (UNICEF 2021). Since low educational attainment correlates with lower earnings, these children are likely to end up in the same position as their parents. In contrast, people with a high income can afford devices and human resources that facilitate autonomy and economic self-sufficiency, granting them time and energy to pursue activities outside of work. This ability correlates to better health and the ability to provide their children with a good education. The cycle of poverty or wealth manifests in intergenerational health and wealth outcomes.

Human resources: Macro-level issues

As described above, people develop personal capabilities through their activities. Since the range of available and accessible activities can be limited by large-scale practices, such as wars, corrupt political practices and unfair competition, certain communities find themselves with limited opportunities to develop personal capabilities, even if some individuals within the community do have a strong capability set. In many countries, there is a drift away from the countryside and into the cities, as people seek better opportunities for themselves and their families. Once people have acquired an education, they may be reluctant to move to rural areas where there is less possibility of professional development and advancement. It follows that certain places, such as deep rural locations and the slum areas of large cities, are more impoverished in terms of human resources than more attractive or affluent locations; and those people who do manage to develop their capabilities are unlikely to choose to stay in a deprived area.

Those occupational therapists who choose to work in remote rural areas, war zones, natural disaster areas and other places on the margins may find them difficult to access, due to poor transport and communication infrastructures. Bringing together human resources in the right place at the right time requires the support of large organisations, such as governments and international aid agencies, who can provide specialised transport, security, space and consumables for healthcare. Local people are needed to provide information and broker access to communities, creating a bridge between the macro-resources of large organisations and the micro-level of the people in need.

A final issue to consider is how the values and goals of large-scale political, economic and social practices can be used to recruit human resources to support the occupational therapist's work. This might be done through developing strategies to enact national policies in practice (Lorenzo 2016), as was illustrated in Case study 1 in Chapter 6.

Micro-level resource issues in diverse settings

Many of the diverse settings where occupational therapists work are termed 'low-resource', meaning there is limited funding, few human resources providing services and little or none of the equipment or materials found in mainstream therapeutic settings. With ingenuity, however, every environment is rich in potential resources. The therapist has to examine the human and non-human elements in the setting to determine which of them are potential resources and how they can be used (Creek 2014). Micro-resources are explored in four categories: personal capabilities, material resources, space-time and human resources. Each of these categories is discussed from a practice theory perspective in relation to occupational performance and occupational therapy practice in diverse, marginalised settings. However, it should be recognised that this categorisation is a convenient simplification of the multiplicity of different types of resources that are an integral part of occupational performance, and of the interrelationships between resources.

This section begins with a case study describing the work of an occupational therapist with displaced persons that is then used to illustrate how resources are identified, utilised and maximised within a particular setting.

Case study 1: CircusAid, by Jill Maglio

CircusAid started when founder Jill Maglio, licensed and registered occupational therapist, walked into a refugee camp in Greece and saw refugees void of occupation and joy due to the deprivation of living in tents without plumbing and with limited basic necessities. There was nothing for people to do on a daily basis but wait for information about their asylum cases. Their immediate and long-term future was uncertain and some had been there for months. What started as a short circus performance, for the promotion of social interaction and artistic expression, transformed into a social enterprise to aid communities displaced by conflict and natural disaster internationally, by giving them autonomy in activities they choose to do and thus promoting a process of healthy development and occupational expression (Maglio and McKinstry 2008).

CircusAid continues to work in refugee camps in Greece and in communities displaced by natural disaster in Indonesia, bringing programmes that combine occupational therapy and circus arts to address the occupational and well-being needs of displaced persons. Grounded in occupational therapy theory and practice and social circus research and practice (Maglio and McKinstry 2008), CircusAid collaborates with local organisations to deliver programmes that promote mental health, community connection and the acquisition of relevant life skills needed to thrive in places of resettlement and life thereafter. Relevant life skills include socialisation, creative thinking, problem-solving and positive risk-taking (CircusAid.com).

Identifying resources: Places and people

In response to the refugee crisis that began in 2015, with conflicts in a number of Middle Eastern countries, Greek authorities constructed refugee camps to house asylum seekers who arrived on European shores seeking refuge. These refugees lived in tents and containers for months and years, without the right to work or freedom of movement. Conditions in the camps were dangerous due to overcrowding, extreme weather, lack of resources and limited health and safety measures; in addition to the presence of children and adults with untreated, complex trauma and constant risk of assault and exploitation. In the camps, people lacked purposeful activity; the occupations they had prior to fleeing their home countries were disrupted in many areas, including work, education and self-care, as well as roles in the family and community.

After building her experience by running short programmes in refugee camps, Jill was able to advocate for her CircusAid project. Demonstrating understanding of the context and population, she approached the managers of Greek refugee camps to promote what CircusAid could offer to the residents there and what logistical supports and permissions were needed to run a month-long programme. Jill established agreements with humanitarian organisations in the camps and coordinated partnerships. She then found interested volunteers, who heard about the project via word-of-mouth and social media. At a later stage, Jill was able to act as a fieldwork supervisor and take on occupational therapy students.

A typical CircusAid programme includes morning training for volunteers and afternoon programmes with children in the camp. Partner organisations at the camp send groups of children to participate according to age or ability. The programme runs for two to three hours a day, two to three days a week in each camp.

The most important resources for Jill to identify initially were the location and the partners. Flexibility is crucial in the context of a refugee camp, with a population (including the staff of NGOs) experiencing ongoing stress and a lack of physical and personal resources.

CircusAid's priority is impact-focused, meaning staff at times act with minimal resources because the true essence of the work is carried out through human resources. It is still possible to have an impact with less people and resources than what is an ideal scenario. The impact of the work really comes down to showing up, presence and clearly wanting to be there to play. All the other materials and equipment are the tools used to engage with the people the team are working with.

Utilising resources: Volunteers

The work of CircusAid relies on a diverse group of volunteers, supporters and partner organisations. Prepared volunteers are the most valuable resource; while unprepared volunteers are the biggest drain on resources. In order to recruit the best fit, volunteers are asked to identify what their individual strengths are and how they want to contribute. If there is congruency with the project's overarching goals and objectives, they are invited to join and co-create a unique experience. Volunteers from the field of occupational therapy are students, recent graduates or people considering occupational therapy as a career, who want experience. Volunteers with an occupational therapy background provide a more therapeutic approach to the project, while volunteers with more circus skills provide performance skills.

A prepared volunteer is able to work as part of a team (demonstrating communication, reliability and accountability) and prioritise the collective goals. When a project is clearly constructed and communication channels with stakeholders are functioning well, CircusAid is able to deliver a powerful experience for participants, volunteers and partners that supports social cohesion and trauma recovery (see CircusAid Methodology for explanation). In four years of practice, CircusAid has worked with over 100 volunteers.

Maximising resources: Adaptation

Continual problem-solving is part of the job when working in an unstable situation. Adaptability is a major strength. CircusAid has performed in parking lots, classrooms, containers and other spaces within Greece, often having to respond quickly to unexpected obstacles, like shifts in permissions to enter camps or cancellations in partnerships.

Funds are required to build infrastructure and secure high-quality material resources. Jill created an advisory board as a resource for business decisions. In addition to funding resources of family, friends and small fundraisers, Jill began to require volunteers to raise money to support their participation. She learned along the way that the CircusAid daily programme is only as strong as her weakest volunteer. By asking volunteers to fundraise for their role, she increased their accountability and commitment, while sustaining the programme. To ensure that volunteers are emotionally stable and bring the appropriate energy, she gives them guidance, preparation and supervision.

Table 7.2 Resources utilised by CircusAid

Personal capabilities

Humanity and integrity; respect for self and others, self-awareness, accountability, willingness to listen, communicate and work towards collective goals with multiple stakeholders.

Planning and project management skills.

Being able to see the full picture and how the different parts relate.

Material resources

Accommodation, transportation.

CircusAid dome, circus equipment, training methods, curriculums, evaluation methods and information packets.

Funds and donations.

Space-time

Flat space, like a field or parking lot, that can fit 15–30 people.

Geodesic dome to create physical space for activities.

Sessions are up to two hours, two to three times a week.

Three months of project planning yearly.

Human resources

Persons who are willing to show up, learn, process, be accountable and contribute funding. Volunteers, skilled local labour, funders, advisors and partners.

CircusAid participants, partner organisations, volunteers/students, funders, community representatives and local labour to help in the setup and material production.

She says that the team's job is to bring joy, which also means sharing and taking on some pain and trauma. Fragility does not really work in this environment. It needs to be processed, grounded, compartmentalised, whatever people need to do to deal with their own emotional response so they can show up ready to play, to bring joy and connect. That is the job of CircusAid: to bring happiness and healing through presence and movement. It is the staff's responsibility to take care of themselves so they can do that.

Each project demands continued collaboration, flexibility and focus on the needs of every community served by CircusAid. Partners and volunteers must have this same vision to ensure that the programme is successful in bringing the joyful and therapeutic experience of circus to large, displaced populations in Greece.

The resources from Case study 1 are displayed in Table 7.2, in the four resource categories.

Personal capabilities: Micro-level issues

As described in the introduction, personal capabilities are the embodied pre-conditions that enable a person to engage in the performance of occupations (Kuijer, Nicenboim and Giaccardi 2017). On a micro-level, these pre-conditions include competences, meanings and motivations. Personal resources are often intangible but nevertheless crucial to the performance of any occupation, especially those that present challenges. These resources reflect the individual's experience of interaction with the world (Kuijer, Nicenboim and Giaccardi 2017) and have been shaped by social and physical contexts. A therapist going to work in an unfamiliar context will gradually develop new and more relevant competences with experience.

The professional competences of an occupational therapist include professional knowledge, clinical and professional reasoning, communication skills, grading tasks, and understanding of documentation processes; but can also mean budgeting, planning and computer skills. Personal competences include personal skills and knowledge, such as awareness of one's own limitations; internal strengths and capacities, such as acceptance of the capacities and limitations of others, and the mental ability to solve problems, lead and draw upon prior experience. Additional personal competences that support practice in marginal settings include flexibility, responsiveness, creativity, openness, assertiveness, intuition, leadership, entrepreneurship and co-operativeness. All these personal and professional competences were illustrated in Case study 1.

Each partner or team member in a project brings their own capabilities and limitations. Where human resources are scarce, it is important for effective team-working to both develop people's competences and accommodate their limitations, as described in Box 7.5.

Box 7.5   Accommodating the abilities and needs of team members

The occupational therapist working in a community setting may find that some of the partners in a project do not espouse professional values but they can still be useful team members. The team have to work with what each person can do, rather than excluding them for what they are not able to do. For example, an occupational therapist taking a job in a marginalised setting found himself working with people who had stolen from the employing organisation. The team recognised that it would be a mistake to put these people into situations where they would be exposed to further opportunities for stealing but, at the same time, supported them to work through their shame. The limitation to this approach comes where an individual's actions might endanger other people or the project.

Some people make fairly large mistakes at work, especially when moving to an unfamiliar setting, and many are able to learn through them. Opportunities to gain experience and learn from one's errors can therefore be seen as a type of resource. For example, a therapist working with street children might have to endure having their personal possessions stolen, until they learn how to keep them safe. Stealing may be necessary for survival but it may also be related to the performance of identity, which is shaped by the meaning of activity, social understandings and engagement in social rules that might not have been part of the therapist's background. How the therapist responds to this experience can be a test of whether or not they will be able to tolerate working in that community. Making a big fuss about such losses could be unproductive and lead to the therapist being excluded.

Relationships are the central resource for occupational therapists and for anyone in a health or helping profession whose basic requirement for successful intervention starts with the client connection. Having the ability to engage with people from diverse backgrounds, in different settings, understanding that everyone's worldview and past experiences differ, is known as *relational agency* (Edwards 2005). In marginalised populations and diverse contexts, like refugee camps, the experienced therapist must bring humility, understanding and patience, especially if there is a likelihood of being viewed as an outsider. The therapist needs to be aware that a group or community may have had negative experiences with other healthcare practitioners. It is not enough for the therapist to prove that she is qualified or licensed to practise; such qualifications may not have any meaning to potential participants.

What a person chooses to do is shaped by the social and personal meanings of the chosen activity, which include its goal, or purpose, and the beliefs, emotions and moods associated with it (Schatzki 1996). Both these dimensions, goal-orientation and affect, contribute to the social meaning of an occupation and to the meaning of each particular performance. For example, there is an interaction between social understandings of what constitutes acceptable occupational therapy practice and how the therapist brings together and utilises available resources to create acceptable performance in context. At first, it may appear there is a lack of resources in the setting, with which to achieve therapeutic goals, especially if the available resources are not the ones she is familiar with. She must be creative and adaptable to work out how best to make use of what is there.

The occupational therapist may draw on personal resources without awareness or acknowledgement of their presence (Creek 2014). An example of an unacknowledged personal resource is the ability to produce flexible and innovative responses when faced with barriers to accessing people and space. This is seen in Case study 1, where the therapist thinks on her feet, uses her previous experience to generate potential solutions, communicates with stakeholders and gatekeepers about her offering and then takes action. She may identify available external resources, such as colleagues and funding, but these solutions are prefigured by the therapist's personal resources of problem-solving and determination.

From a social practice theory perspective, occupational therapy uses the meaning of an activity as a resource as much as material resources; and the cultural meaning of a space is also a resource. Circus can be seen as a cultural space; combining this with the meanings that occupational therapy brings into the place of performance creates something new in the experience people are having. Relational agency within the imaginary spaces of circus practice, combined with the supportive presence of the therapist, creates a safe space in which people feel free to play. Participants of all levels of ability are able to experience success when the community supports participation and positive risk-taking. For example, a child who drops a spinning plate is still celebrated for trying.

Any space can become an imaginary space for play, or for circus as a developed form of play, and the therapist's ability to create this shared space is a crucial competence. The circus becomes a transformational space where reality is suspended for the duration of the performance, in an unspoken contract between performer and audience. The transformational nature of the circus is inherent in the performance as a relationship: the role of the audience is to witness the suspended reality of the performance and the impossible or surreal moment of the action, such as clowning or plate-spinning.

Material resources: Micro-level issues

All occupations are associated with particular material resources; for example, juggling requires three or more balls or other suitable objects. However, each performance of an occupation can utilise materials available in the environment as resources; for example, an improvised juggling practice can use dried banana leaves tied into balls.

In order to utilise local resources, the therapist has to become familiar with what is available from communities, corporations, health systems and other organisations. This often requires reaching out, networking and communicating with others, including healthcare professionals, charities, local government bodies and industry leaders, who may provide access to various types of material resources. Access to workspaces and to tools required to do therapy is often negotiated by therapists. For example, an occupational therapist wants to start working with children with special needs who come into a community centre. If the service area is not an established space for occupational therapy, there will be no standardised tools or play therapy equipment and the therapist has to find or create her own. In this situation, the therapist can improvise, using whatever materials are available in the environment. The therapist might also ask peers and colleagues, other therapy clinics, her university and the local community to donate equipment and lend assessment forms.

Money is an essential resource for occupational therapy practice, both for reimbursing staff and for buying equipment and materials. Many occupational therapists who work in diverse settings have to apply for their own grants or find partners to collaborate with in order to fund a position or project. Economic resourcefulness requires the skills of managing funds and budgeting. For example, in Case study 1, when funding was scarce, the therapist incorporated occupational therapy student fieldwork into the project so that she could be reimbursed for her role as a supervisor, using this money to support the programme.

Space-time: Micro-level issues

Occupational therapy practice is always located within space-time, in that everything the therapist does involves a doing-place, a historical context, a time for intervention and a future orientation (Schatzki 1996; Shove, Pantzar and Watson 2012). The actions and performances of the therapist and others co-exist and co-evolve within particular social spaces and times (Dreier 2008).

The occupational therapist has to consider how resources can be identified, brought together and utilised within the structured, physical space and the abstract space-time of the place for intervention; and this organisation might have to be negotiated with the community. For example, in Case study 1, the therapist had to negotiate an appropriate space in the refugee camp for the activities to take place that was accessible and could be reserved for the intended audience.

Providing safe spaces for therapeutic interventions is an essential aspect of good practice. This includes a structured place where people can feel physically safe but also a mental space in which people feel their identities and contributions to the experience are not under threat. The resourceful occupational therapist is able to create space and time for intervention that appeals to the target group and promotes occupational participation and functional recovery, however, limited the progress might be.

Time is a resource that often seems simple until different elements of individual and community realities become apparent. The experienced therapist recognises that a pragmatic approach may be necessary when organising interventions that require people to commit their time, and this applies to both participants and staff. Working with low-income or marginalised communities necessitates flexibility with regard to schedules and the timing of appointments. For example, in the CircusAid programme for trauma recovery, allocating an hour for a training does not take account of the initial socialisation that may be necessary to create a therapeutic environment, allow for delays in people getting to the group or leave time for planning future activities. Also, it may be important to think about the time of day that appointments are made for persons who have survived trauma or those from different cultures. Stress and difficulties with transport can influence attendance in community-based settings. Interventions and projects are likely to proceed more smoothly if the voice of participants is heard with regard to their timing and length.

There is a distinct need for informal social spaces to encourage trust-building and bonding with any newcomers, again reflecting cultural space. This bonding needs to occur in a short time and space in order for participants to learn new skills or construct new performances. However, community networking over time may be essential for communities to build trust and invest themselves into the project. Making time for these informal social spaces also supports getting buy-in and honest feedback from participants with regard to the service offered, which are essential for the sustainability of the projects.

The future aspect of space-time is expressed in terms of the objectives, goals and aspirations of the therapist and everyone else involved in the project. All human action is future-oriented, in that people do things with certain objectives in mind. When the occupational therapist plans a cooking group, she has reasons for doing so, for example, because she wants to encourage social interaction between participants; because participants want to learn how to cook with unfamiliar ingredients; because someone needs to make dinner for the participants, or because participants have asked for an opportunity to cook for pleasure. Participants in the cookery group have their own reasons for participating, which may have little to do with the therapist's objectives. The practice of cooking itself follows a certain progression through time, from ingredients to the meal. In order for the activity to be performed in such a way that it is recognisable as cooking, it proceeds step-by-step towards a future goal, in a sequence that is socially accepted as cooking a meal.

Human resources: Micro-level issues

Human resources for occupational therapy practice include not only the numbers of people who might potentially participate but also their competences, their willingness to be used as resources and their availability in the right place at the right time.

Potential human resources may be participants, colleagues, managers, students, families, neighbours, peers and many others. The trust and understanding of all these people are essential to recruit them into a project. When therapists are tasked with acquiring new staff or volunteers, or with finding partners for a project, they must understand the number of people needed, the desired skills and the motivations required. If the skills and motivations of recruits do not match the needs of the project, there is a risk that volunteers or paid staff become liabilities rather than resources. An example of this is seen in Case study 1, where the therapist came to depend on the numbers and the quality of her volunteers to be able to sustain the project. The therapist needs to have a clear vision of what she is trying to achieve and ensure that any potential partners both understand it and are prepared to support it.

People's reasons for participating in a project will include both the purpose it has for them and how they feel about it (Schatzki 1996). In order to recruit participants, therefore, the occupational therapist has to have a clear understanding of how members of the community understand their own needs, what their goals are, who is responsible for their well-being and what they expect to gain from participation. Ideally, the occupational therapist is given enough time and space to embed themselves sufficiently to reach this understanding. In reality, they are often expected to take immediate action and may have to work through participants' disappointment when they find their expectations of occupational therapy to be misaligned.

In settings that have limited material resources, different human resources may be required and may shape the goals and processes of therapist and client. Taking a pragmatic approach enables the therapist to adapt her practice to the resources available. For example, a hospital or well-funded home setting is likely to be provisioned with material resources that facilitate a range of future-oriented possibilities. On the other hand, a community setting may be rich in human resources but be relatively limited in terms of its material affordances. The therapist may need to recruit a particular set of human resources in order to use the materials at hand in pursuit of future goals. This point is explored further in the next section.

Resourcefulness

One of the most important capabilities for occupational therapists working in diverse settings is resourcefulness. 'Resourcefulness occurs in situations that are in some way exceptional, non-standard, non-routine or non-mainstream' (Kuijer, Nicenboim and Giaccardi 2017: 18). The occupational therapist engages human and non-human resources in therapy and, in doing so, helps clients and co-workers discover how to find and utilise resources for themselves. Part of the role of the therapist is to share ways of performing practices that people might take up and use themselves, by knowing when to step back and let other people feel they are in control. When accustomed resources are not readily available, the therapist needs to have the ability to see people and things that are there in the environment as potential resources and to visualise how they might be used.

What is resourcefulness?

Resourcefulness is the name given to the 'practices by which users adapt, repurpose, and appropriate existing artefacts from their surroundings' (Kuijer, Nicenboim and Giaccardi 2017: 17). It involves a complex interplay between the purpose of an action and the means by which it can be performed, through which both purpose and means are reconfigured to create a fit.

Resourcefulness requires ingenuity, improvisation and self-reliance. The capability to identify and utilise a wide range of resources is an essential skill that occupational therapists must develop in order to work effectively in diverse and poorly resourced settings. Where there is a lack of familiar material and human resources, an ability to adapt and improvise allows for alternative ways of using what is there. An example of improvising with material resources is appropriate paper-based technology (APT), which is used to make low-cost, specialised seating and other equipment (Kingsley 2010). An example of improvising with human resources is teaching family members to become co-therapists in the treatment and rehabilitation of disabled people (Grossman and Shuma 2010).

Personal capacities can sometimes act as barriers to resourcefulness. For example, resistance to demonstrating vulnerability may restrict the therapist from asking for help; or believing that practice should be guided by systematised frameworks may restrict the therapist from thinking outside commonly used approaches and models for practice. The original design of artefacts can also make it easier or more difficult for the therapist to envisage alternative uses or ways of utilising them. For example, a cooking pot can be used to carry water, boil water, cook food or dye cloth, whereas an electric kettle was designed to boil water and is less adaptable to other purposes. The cooking pot can be used with a variety of fuel sources while the electric kettle requires an electricity supply. We could say that the design of the electric kettle imposes its meaning on the user while a cooking pot allows for multiple interpretations (Kuijer, Nicenboim and Giaccardi 2017).

Case study 2 describes one therapist's transition from mainstream health services into a community-based setting, requiring vision and ingenuity in order to identify, utilise and maximise resources that were not readily available. It is possible to identify in this case study some of the components of resourcefulness described above.

Case study 2: Occupational therapy in primary care

A local NHS mental health trust had funding to set up a mental health occupational therapy service in a general practice located on a socially and economically deprived housing estate in the northeast of England. The housing estate was physically run-down, with only a small number of shops and poor transport links to the city centre. The estate was therefore relatively isolated within the region and many of the residents did not travel outside the estate very often.

The primary care setting employed two general practitioners (GPs), several nurses, a health visitor, a community dietician and a community psychiatric nurse (CPN). Lauren, an occupational therapist with 15 years of experience in conventional adult mental health settings, was contracted to work two days a week for 18 months and was required to work independently.

Lauren was challenged when she found that the CPN received all mental health referrals and there were no opportunities for her to deliver occupational therapy services. She decided to try to engage the local community by visiting local community centres, children's nurseries and mental health charities to talk about her role. After she explained to each organisation what occupational therapy services she could offer, they invited her to work with them: eventually, what started as an 18-month project lasted for over five years.

With the permission of the head occupational therapist and the lead GP, Lauren took over a women's craft group in a local community centre. The community workers had observed that many of the women had mental health problems they did not have the skills to address. The GP saw this as a mental health promotion opportunity: if Lauren could increase the women's emotional resilience, they would be better able to cope with the problems of everyday life and less likely to seek medical intervention for minor issues.

In order to advertise the group to community members, the centre did a leaflet drop around the estate, describing an initial six craft sessions. These were designed to be three-hours long, every Monday morning, with a different craft taught each week. The community centre provided a room with suitable furniture for the group to use and a small budget for materials, which Lauren sourced from cheap stores and charity shops.

This was Lauren's first experience of mental health promotion and she began with a literature search for evidence of community-based interventions shown to increase people's ability to overcome adverse life events. From accounts of these interventions, she was able to develop strategies that she built into the craft sessions; for example, a tea break was incorporated into each session to encourage social interaction and network-building.

Staff at the community centre were satisfied with the success of the women's group and asked Lauren to become involved in other projects. One of these was a school holiday play scheme for children on the estate. Staff ran a variety of activity groups in local primary schools so that children had something constructive to do during the day. Lauren ran craft sessions for large groups of children, helping them to develop basic skills, such as paying attention, following instructions, taking turns and sharing.

The biggest resource challenge for Lauren was gaining access to the target client group when her expectations for referrals at the GP practice were not met. She had to network, articulate what occupational therapy could offer the community and advertise her services. In looking for innovative ways of accessing the target group, she drew on her own adaptability, ingenuity and commitment. This resourcefulness led to various offers of opportunities to work. In describing this process, Lauren said:

> Do not be defensive or apologetic about what you have to offer. If people say they do not understand your role, show them what you can do. If people say that what you do is common sense and anyone could do it, invite them to work with you. Team-working is essential in a community setting.

Lauren's personality and people skills were paramount to working effectively in a low-income, community-based mental health setting, where her education and accent initially set her apart from the people she wanted to work with. She observed:

> When I started working on the housing estate, the gap between my life experiences and those of the residents looked as though it could be a barrier. However, we were able to build warm, mutually respectful relationships through working together ... We chose not to judge each other but to learn about and from each other.

When the 18-month NHS contract expired, Lauren continued to run groups in the community centre and other venues on the estate, thanks to European Union funding. She worked there part-time for a further four years, facilitating groups for primary school children, adolescents and older people, in addition to the women's group. Crucial to the success and sustained impact of the occupational therapy service was the creation of strong therapeutic relationships with clients. Lauren spoke of how she learned to adapt to a new way of working:

> The most important things I learned were that there is no captive audience when you are doing community work and that you have to be flexible, open and responsive to what is happening. When I made mistakes, people did not return to my groups. I rapidly learned what was needed and how to provide it in ways that were acceptable to participants.

Another key factor was Lauren's ability to build mutually supportive, trusting relationships with staff in the general practice and at the community centre. All of Lauren's work came through these people so the success of the project depended on her relationships with them. She noted that: 'Partnership working and clear communication were essential to the success of this project'.

Lauren invested her time and energy in the community: her commitment and flexibility, together with interpersonal skills and ingenuity, enabled her to offer services to many different groups in the community and ensured the continuation of a funded occupational therapy role. Many years of experience as a practising occupational therapist gave Lauren the confidence to extend into new roles, such as mental health promotion, without overstepping her professional boundaries. She emphasised the importance of professional confidence:

> It is important to be confident in your professional role and skills so that you are comfortable deciding what is within your remit and where you will need support. Feeling anxious and insecure can lead to defensiveness and setting rigid boundaries, which are unproductive in marginal settings. When you go into an unfamiliar, under-resourced situation, accept that you do not immediately know what to do and take time to learn as much as you can before acting. Seek feedback in any form and from anyone. Above all, avoid imposing prior expectations and structures on unfamiliar situations: doing so will block your capacity to learn.

The goal of occupational therapy in this setting was to encourage people in the community to change their social practices in ways that would benefit their health. Lauren did not try to change people's behaviour but worked to create circumstances in which they would recognise their own capacity for change and retain ownership of their practices.

Summary and conclusion

This chapter employed a practice theory perspective to explore some of the resource issues that arise in diverse settings. From this perspective, the focus of attention is not the performer or the context of performance but the occupation itself. The chapter started with the premise that human and material resources are integral elements of occupations, which come together in space and time during the occupational performance.

We have seen how practices that influence resource availability and utilisation work on two levels: macro and micro. Macro-level influences operate through social patterns, such as systematised inequality, and social institutions, such as politics. Micro-level issues are situated in particular places and times; meaning that the field of possibilities for action is specific to particular contexts. This point was illustrated through two case studies: one describing the work of an occupational therapist in refugee camps and the other an occupational therapist establishing a mental health service in a primary care setting.

Many of the diverse settings where occupational therapists work are characterised by a lack of familiar human and non-human resources. The therapist has to be able to identify potential resources, find ways to utilise them and maximise their utility. The capability to identify and utilise unfamiliar resources is called *resourcefulness*, which was defined as the ability to adapt, repurpose and appropriate existing artefacts for new uses.

Practitioners working in diverse settings draw on a wide range of professional and personal capabilities in engaging the people and things in the environment for therapeutic purposes. They tend to be pragmatic, responsive, flexible and confident in their professional role. This way of working does not suit everyone; many occupational therapists look for structure and predictability in their daily work. Nonetheless, in a world of rapid and extreme change, there is likely to be an increasing demand for resourceful practitioners who can adapt their practice to suit non-traditional settings.

The next chapter explores the nature of change and how occupational therapists can adapt to meet the shifting health and social care demands of the modern world.

References

Abramsky, S. (2013) *The American way of poverty: how the other half still lives*. New York: Nation Books.

Blue, S., Shove, E., Carmona, C., and Kelly, M.P. (2014) Theories of practice and public health: understanding (un)healthy practices. *Critical Public Health*, 26(1): 36–50.

CircusAid Methodology (2020) Online at https://www.circusaid.com/hct-methodolgy. Accessed December 2020.

Creek, J. (2014) *Transformative occupational therapy practice: learning from the margins* (Doctoral dissertation, University of Sheffield, The School of Education).

Dreier, O. (2008) *Psychotherapy in everyday life*. Cambridge: Cambridge University Press.

Edwards, A. (2005) Relational agency: learning to be a resourceful practitioner. *International Journal of Educational Research*, 43(3): 168–182.

Grossman, H., and Shuma, B.E. (2010) Occupational therapy in mentally and physically challenged children – a model for East Africa based on the Tanzania experience. In: V. Alers and R. Crouch (eds.) *Occupational therapy: an African perspective*. Johannesburg: Sarah Shorten. 156–169.

Hui, A., and Walker, G. (2018) Concepts and methodologies for a new relational geography of energy demand: social practices, doing-places and settings. *Energy Research and Social Science*, 36: 21–29.

Kingsley, F. (2010) Fabrication and production of low cost aids and adapted equipment. In: V. Alers, and R. Crouch (eds.) *Occupational therapy: an African perspective*. Johannesburg: Sarah Shorten. 134–154.

Kuijer, L., Nicenboim, I., and Giaccardi, E. (2017) Conceptualising resourcefulness as a dispersed practice. In: *Proceedings of the 2017 Conference on Designing Interactive Systems*. 15–27.

Lorenzo, T. (2016) Political reasoning for disability inclusion: making policies practical. In: M. Cole and J. Creek (eds.) *Global perspectives in professional reasoning*. New Jersey: Slack. 77–98.

Maglio, J., and McKinstry, C. (2008) Occupational therapy and circus: potential partners in enhancing the health and well-being of today's youth. *Australian Occupational Therapy Journal*, 55(4): 287–290.

Nicolini, D. (2012) *Practice theory, work and organization: an introduction*. Oxford: Oxford University Press.

Norman, D.A. (2013) *The design of everyday things, revised and expanded edition*. Cambridge, MA: MIT Press.

OECD (2013) *Survey of adult skills*. Online at www.oecd.org/skills/piaac/Countrynote-United Kingdom.pdf. Accessed May 2022.

Reckwitz, A. (2002) Towards a theory of social practices: a development in cultural theorizing. *European Journal of Social Theory*, 5(2): 243–263.

Røpke, I. (2009) Theories of practice – new inspiration for ecological economic studies on consumption. *Ecological Economics*, 68: 2490–2497.

Schatzki, T.R. (2001) Introduction: practice theory. In: T.R. Schatzki, K. Knorr Cetina and E. von Savigny (eds.) *The practice turn in contemporary theory*. London: Routledge. 10–23.

Schatzki, T.R. (1996) *Social practices: a Wittgensteinian approach to human activity and the social*. Cambridge: Cambridge University Press.

Sen, A. (1999) *Development as freedom*. Oxford: Oxford University Press.

Shorter Oxford English Dictionary (2002) *Shorter Oxford English Dictionary*. Oxford: Oxford University Press.

Shove, E. (2017) Matters of practice. In: A. Hui, T. Schatzki and E. Shove (eds.) *The nexus of practices: connections, constellations, practitioners*. London: Routledge. 155–168.

Shove, E., Pantzar, M., and Watson, M. (2012) *The dynamics of social practice: everyday life and how it changes*. Los Angeles: Sage.

UNICEF (2019) *Literacy*. Online at https://data.unicef.org/topic/education/literacy/. Accessed May 2022.

UNICEF (2021) *Child labour*. Online at https://www.unicef.org/protection/child-labour Accessed May 2022.

Watson, M. (2017) Placing power in practice theory. In: A. Hui, T. Schatzki and E. Shove (eds.) *The nexus of practices: connections, constellations, practitioners*. London: Routledge. 169–182.

8   Change in occupational therapy

*Ana Carreira De Mello, Taís Quevedo Marcolino,
and Nick Pollard*

With acknowledgements to Francis Ekwan

Introduction

Change has been a constant throughout human history, although some things change
more quickly than others. Social changes can take place suddenly, such as the invasion
of Ukraine by Russia in 2022, whereas geological changes tend to happen slowly, for
example, the erosion of rocks. The 21st century has seen an acceleration of the pace of
change on a global scale, in areas such as:

- the demographic make-up of society, with an increase in the proportion of older
  people;
- technological advances, such as digital banking;
- political shifts, including the rise of populism;
- climate and environmental changes, leading to more frequent and severe natural
  disasters;
- socio-economic developments, including an expanding gap between rich and
  poor.

These changes affect many social practices, such as facilitating new practices and
obviating the need for others. For example, the invention of the internal combustion
engine and the motor car gave a new level of freedom of movement to many people
but caused such trades as blacksmiths, grooms, and farriers to become redundant.

This chapter begins with a discussion of what change is and how it occurs, using a
practice theory perspective. The change process is illustrated with an example of
changing practices in community healthcare in the United Kingdom. The second
section explores how macro-level issues influence the development and performance of
occupational therapy, using the example of how the profession developed in Brazil.
The third section takes three case studies from Brazil to show how change occurs at
the micro-level through occupational therapy intervention.

What is change and how does it occur?

There are many ways of understanding change, from a painful inevitability to an
opportunity that can be seized. The Shorter Oxford English Dictionary (2002) defined
change as 'making or becoming different; alteration in state or quality; mutation'.
Some philosophers have associated the concept of change with the concept of an **event**;
'an event is a change in some object or other' (Audi 1999: 293). Practice theorists

DOI: 10.4324/9781003016755-8

conceptualise **time** as 'the flow and pace of events' (Chapter 3: XX), indicating that change occurs in space-time. An event may be of limited duration, for example, switching on a light, or may take place over an extended period, for example, sailing around the world. Whatever the length of time taken, an event produces a change in the material world, such as lighting a room or moving a person from one place to another.

A practice exists as an entity, independent of when and how it is performed; for example, we can talk about the practice of cooking without having to think about specific instances of cooking. A practice 'exists as a recognizable conjunction of *elements* [e.g. kitchen, utensils, ingredients, recipes, bodily competences, purposes], consequently figuring as an *entity* which can be spoken about and more importantly drawn upon as a set of resources when [cooking]' (Shove et al. 2012: 7). A practice persists in space-time through repeated performances, with each performance differing in context, performer, meaning and so on. For example, cooking performances in rural Zambia and urban New York consist of different spaces, equipment, ingredients, methods, performers and purposes. In turn, the practice-as-entity changes over time, through an accumulation of differences in performance. The process of change is not linear; often there are interruptions and further changes that affect the direction and pace of change. Once a dynamic change is released, like a snooker ball making the first break, the change interacts with other elements, precipitating further changes.

Shove and colleagues (2012) explored the mechanisms by which practices persist and change; including how they emerge, exist and disappear, and how multiple practices coalesce, combine and separate. They began the process of understanding change with a simple scheme describing practices in terms of three elements: materials, competences and meanings. **Materials** include 'things, technologies, tangible physical entities, and the stuff of which objects are made' (Shove et al. 2012: 14). **Competences** encompass 'skill, know-how and techniques' (Shove et al. 2012: 14). **Meanings** include 'symbolic meanings, ideas, and aspirations' (Shove et al. 2012: 14). The elements of cooking are outlined in Box 8.1.

Box 8.1   The elements of cooking as a practice

The practice of cooking consists of a dynamic amalgam of materials, competences, and meanings. The particular conjunction of elements varies from one performance to another, but the practice is always recognisable as cooking.

The **materials** of cooking include the *space*, such as a kitchen; *artefacts*, such as a stove, *infrastructure*, such as a water supply, and *consumable resources*, such as ingredients. The body of the cook can also be seen as a material element.

The **competences** of cooking include *knowledge*, such as how ingredients are changed by different cooking processes; *know-how*, such as how to prepare ingredients, and *skills*, such as using a sharp knife safely.

The **meaning** of cooking includes *purposes*, such as producing a meal for the family, *beliefs*, such as celebrating a birthday, *emotions*, such as pride in being a good cook, and *motivation*, such as hunger.

A practice-as-entity consists of an integrated set of elements that relate to each other in some way. For example, cooking involves some combination of the materials, competences and meanings described in Box 8.1. Practice-as-performance varies because the elements combine in different ways on different occasions. Through examining the three elements that make up a practice, we can see that a change in any of these elements affects how the practice is performed. For example, when a house is connected to an electricity supply (materials), meals can be cooked indoors on an electric stove rather than outside over an open fire. Having access to a good recipe book enables the cook to extend her repertoire of dishes for the family (competences). If a family decides to stop eating meat, fish, and dairy produce (meanings), different ingredients and processes are needed to produce vegan dishes. Recipes and cooking methods may be handed down through the generations, often from mother to daughter, but they gradually evolve as different resources become available and tastes change, for example, producing vegan versions of favourites and using substitutes such as jackfruit for meat.

No practice exists in isolation but is always linked to other practices. For example, Blue and Spurling (2017) described a hospital as a complex of connected and interdependent practices that combine in different ways at different times (Box 8.2).

Box 8.2   The hospital as an evolving complex of practices (after Blue and Spurling 2017)

A hospital is the site of multiple practices that combine and coordinate 24 hours a day, 365 days a year; including such activities as surgery, nursing, physiotherapy, visiting, catering, cleaning, record-keeping, dispensing, accounting and many more. All these practices collaborate and compete for time and space and are, in turn, shaped by the spatial-temporal organisation of the hospital.

Over time, the design of hospital buildings evolves to facilitate new practices and new ways of practising, such as the change, in the United Kingdom, from caring for patients in Nightingale wards to single rooms. Technological innovation enables and demands new ways of working across many practices; for example, moving from paper records to electronic record-keeping. Advances in knowledge translate into different goals and methods of treatment, such as getting patients out of bed as soon as possible after surgery to reduce the risk of thrombosis, rather than recommending bed rest. The managerialisation of healthcare services changes the relationships between practices, for example, clinical goals may be determined by managers rather than by doctors (see Chapter 2).

Blue and Spurling (2017) theorised that change in a complex environment, such as a hospital, does not occur within discrete practices themselves but in the interconnections between practices. In their example of the hospital, the life of the institution is transformed across multiple registers, including

... advances in medical science and in theories of infection and disease; a reconfigured and extended system of health professions, with their altered, emergent and redundant jurisdictions and areas of expertise; cultural shifts in social categories like children and childhood, social class, gender and age, all of which have implications for ideas of good hospital care; along with changed schedules and rotas of staff and patients associated with new forms of training, departmental opening hours, and different kinds of treatment, therapy and surveillance.

(Blue and Spurling 2017: 26)

Change in one element of a practice can transform that practice; and change in one practice brings about change in other, related practices. This is now explored using the example of community healthcare.

How change happens in healthcare provision

Changing one element of a healthcare service, whether materials, competences or meanings, can have a major influence on other elements and on the way services develop. Professional practices take advantage of technological innovations but are themselves altered by their use and the profusion of changes that result. For example, in community health services, at one time nurses used bicycles to visit patients at home but later had access to cars to carry out their work (Greenlees 2018). As cars became widely used and economically viable for community nurses, certain healthcare practices were made available to a wider section of the population. Nurses can carry more equipment in a car than on a bicycle, making it possible for patients to have more treatments at home. With the digitisation of records, it became possible for nurses to take laptop computers with them on home visits, for recording and for other functions, meaning that they need not drive back to the office between patients (Abdu and Cooper 2016).

As car use became widespread, driving was added to the skill set of community health professionals; those staff who could not drive were not able to apply for community posts. The introduction of electronic record-keeping meant that staff had to attain at least a basic level of computer literacy to input and access data. These new competences were added to the specialist skills of the healthcare professional.

Changes in the material elements of community healthcare, such as the introduction of cars and computers, have had an impact on what practices can be performed by healthcare professionals, how they are performed and, in turn, the expectations of service providers, professionals themselves and patients. Service providers may see a range of efficiencies in providing cars and computers for community nurses, such as reducing the amount of office space needed. There can also be advantages for professionals in new ways of working. For social workers, the car has been conceptualised as a mobile office, a fluid space in which to process the emotional demands of working with families (Ferguson 2009). The car has become not just a vehicle but also a personal space, in which a practitioner can reflect and prepare between visits (De Certeau 1984). An occupational therapy example of the changing meaning of the car in community practice is given in Box 8.3.

Box 8.3   The meaning of the car in community occupational therapy practice

An occupational therapist in a community mental health team found that car journeys between clients provided time for thinking and preparation. Visits to patients and their families could sometimes be intense in their requirements for observation and negotiation of objectives in the care plan. The interior of the car became a space in which the therapist could engage in micro tactics of restoration; such as playing music, staying in the car to listen to the end of a radio programme, stopping for a sandwich or diverting to enable a visit to a corner shop.

While mobile services may have advantages in health and social care practice, they can also mean that teams meet less, and workers may even lose their team bases altogether. Jeyasingham (2020) explored some of the effects of these developments in child and family social work. For example, communication is often through text and email rather than face-to-face. Written communication can lack the immediacy and nuance of speech and the writer may not know how information is being used by the people who have access to it. Relationships and communications become defined by networks of people who have technical competence or physical access to wifi hotspots, mobile phone coverage or places where they can work on confidential reports. Having facilities for electronic communication and record-keeping may create pressure to see more clients during the working day and, as less time is spent travelling to and from the office, there may be no clear start and finish times. Caseloads increase, leading to further reduction of communication opportunities.

The first section of this chapter described the change process using examples of changing practices in community healthcare in the United Kingdom. The second section explores how macro-level issues influence the development and performance of occupational therapy.

Macro-level influences on change: Occupational therapy in Brazil

This section explores how occupational therapy as a practice entity and practice performance changes over time as other, related social practices change. The development of the profession in Brazil is used to illustrate the processes through which interconnected practices persist and change.

Introduction to Brazil

Brazil is the fifth largest country in the world, in terms of territory; with an area of 8,547,403 km^2 and a population of 214.6 million people (Brazilian Institute of Geography and Statistics [IBGE] 2022). It is divided into 27 states, with populations irregularly distributed across five geographic regions: south, southeast, midwest, north and northeast. Each region includes highly urbanised and industrialised cities, rural areas and uninhabited areas. The largest city in the country, and in the whole of South America, is São Paulo, with 12.39 million inhabitants (IBGE 2022). São Paulo is the capital of the state of São Paulo, the richest in the country. For a long time, it was the state that offered the most job opportunities, which caused a large migration of people from other regions of Brazil, in search of better living conditions.

The Brazilian population has several ethnic groups, including native indigenous populations, Africans brought by slavery and Portuguese groups. Other international migratory movements also occurred and, as a complex and multifactorial phenomenon, contributed to the arrival of Italians, Swiss, Germans and Japanese, among different nationalities that arrived to colonise South America. Thus, the population comprises white, black, brown, mestizo and indigenous peoples (Drummond and Cruz 2018). Brazil is one of the ten most unequal countries in the world, with 55% of the total income going to the richest 10% of the population (UNDP 2019).

From 1964 to 1985, the country lived under the regime of a military dictatorship, which severely compromised the citizenship and rights of Brazilian people. Due to continuing exploitation by the government and multinational corporations, and the struggle to re-democratise the country, civil society organises itself in various movements, such as the student movement, the workers' movement and the movement against hunger, among others. These movements, which began in the era of dictatorship, campaign in the context of a complex of evolving situations, including widespread corruption, claims, counter-claims, and media manipulation, which have at times alienated the public (Drummond and Cruz 2018; Schwarz and Starling 2018; Marques 2020).

Healthcare in Brazil

With the end of the military dictatorship, in the 1980s, the fight for freedom and the re-democratisation process, alongside Brazilian healthcare reform (Escorel 1998), led to the promulgation of the Federal Constitution of 1988 (Brasil 1988), in which health became a citizens' right and a duty of the State. The Constitution also regulates the participation of the private sector in health services, with the commitment that it should be aligned with public policies and subject to state oversight (Machado and Silva 2019).

In this political and social context, the Unified Health System (Sistema Único de Saúde [SUS]) came into being in 1990, on foundations that defended: the democratisation of access to healthcare; the universality of access to healthcare services for all Brazilian citizens, without any discrimination; the quality of services, and equity. The SUS delivers health promotion, preventative actions and curative services at all levels of complexity. This new healthcare model was based on decentralisation and regionalisation, encompassing both actions and health services, and includes primary, medium and high complexity care (Machado and Silva 2019). Box 8.4 illustrates how the principles underpinning the SUS were enacted in the field of mental healthcare.

Box 8.4   The development of mental healthcare in Brazil

In the field of mental health, as part of Brazilian healthcare reforms, the policy was to transform the paradigm of hospital-centred care into community care. This movement was strongly influenced by the mental health service reforms in Italy, which took place between the 1960s and 1970s. Marked by its radicalism, the starting point for the Italian process was a belief that the problems inherent to psychiatric care were the object of political struggle; the aim was social change. This led to demands for the closure of asylums and the transformation of the power relationship between health professionals and their patients (Marques et al. 2020). With the enactment of the Basaglia Law, in 1978, all asylums were closed, giving way to community services. Thus, the process of psychiatric reform in Italy promoted the freedom of patients to live in the community.

The Italian reforms inspired many countries around the world (Serapioni 2019). In Brazil, which Basaglia visited twice, they contributed to the development of practices, theoretical formulations and legislative proposals that had growing resonance. Community psychosocial care was mandated by State policy, with the Ministry of Health responsible for acting (Marques et al. 2020). However, due to economic and political forces, psychiatric hospitals were not entirely abolished in Brazil, as they had been in Italy. Then, in 2001, the Paulo Delgado Law was enacted, which provided for the gradual reduction of psychiatric beds and the expansion of community services (Salles, Barros and Matsukura 2016).

In 2011, the enactment of the Psychosocial Care Network National Policy (RAPS) established a regional network of care points (Fiocruz 2015), with the aim of promoting deinstitutionalisation and psychosocial rehabilitation (Brasil 2013; Salles, Barros, and Matsukura 2016). In fact, the RAPS had been developing gradually since the late 1970s, with the aim of reaching out to people with mental health problems and with issues related to psychoactive substance abuse. The network includes primary care; specialised care services, called Psychosocial Care Centres (CAPS for severe mental disorders; CAPSad for people with drug and alcohol addiction, and CAPSij for children and youth); wards in general hospitals, and specialised wards in psychiatric hospitals.

Since 2002, CAPS have been regulated by the Brazilian Ministry of Health and they are part of the mental healthcare network that replaced the asylum model. Services are provided on an outpatient basis. All the CAPS carry out interdisciplinary psychosocial monitoring of patients and promote social reintegration through access to work, school, leisure and culture, and through seeking to strengthen family and community ties. The service seeks to enable people to progress through significant experiences in mental healthcare towards the exercise of citizenship (Brasil 2004).

CAPSad aims to provide comprehensive care to people who abuse alcohol or are dependent on psychoactive substances, and to their families It also includes a wider range of actions addressed to community and social organisations. It is a specialised service that provides individual care (e.g., medication, psychotherapy, occupational therapy and counselling); group and community care; therapeutic activity groups (such as cooking and theatre); home visits and matrix support actions. Matrix support embraces case discussions and co-responsibility for care between CAPS and primary health teams. CAPSad also carries out early interventions to reduce the stigma associated with treatment (Brasil 2004).

CAPSij provides daily services for the care of severely mentally compromised children and adolescents; including those with autism, psychosis or severe neurosis, and those who have difficulty establishing or maintaining social relationships due to their health conditions (Brasil 2004).

In recent years, neoliberal economic and political forces, in combination with a more conservative movement, have led to community mental healthcare services being gradually dismantled. The treatment of people experiencing mental suffering and those with issues related to the abuse of psychoactive substances is relocating to closed institutions, with a strong religious bias (Lussi et al. 2019).

The history of Brazilian occupational therapy

To date, there is no definitive written history of occupational therapy in Brazil (Melo, 2015).

The account given here takes a historiographical perspective to present and discuss elements of that history. This approach takes time and space as two fundamental variables; contextualising the development of the profession in local experiences and at specific times (Melo 2015).

Between the 1940s and 1960s, some Brazilian psychiatrists, including Nise da Silveira, Ulysses Pernambucano and Luis Cerqueira, recognised the value of therapeutic activities in treating psychiatric conditions and proposed a different approach to intervention (Drummond and Cruz 2018). At the same time as these pioneering initiatives were being established, the country was facing a poliomyelitis epidemic, which highlighted a lack of professionals to provide specialised care for patients (Ferrari 2013). The epidemiological relevance of poliomyelitis was lower than other diseases in this period; however, 60% to 70% of affected children belonged to the higher social classes, thus attracting enough social and political attention to be considered a priority (Barros 2009; Melo 2015). The need was recognised for professionals and technical services to meet emerging demands (Drummond and Cruz 2018).

The United Nations International Movement for Rehabilitation was implemented in Brazil in 1940, when the Institute of Physical Medicine and Rehabilitation was founded at the University of São Paulo (Ferrari 2013). This initiative expanded training and rehabilitation services in the country. Then, in 1951, a few health professionals from the Clinics Hospital of the University of São Paulo went to the United States for specialist training in rehabilitation. One of them was Neyde Tosetti Hauck, a nurse and social worker, who studied occupational therapy at New York University. She became the director of occupational therapy departments at the Clinics Hospital and one of the first occupational therapists to graduate from the University of São Paulo (Soares 1991; Drummond and Cruz 2018).

The first occupational therapy training programme in Brazil was a three-year course, offered in 1956 by the School of Rehabilitation of the Brazilian Beneficent Association for Rehabilitation, in Rio de Janeiro (Barros 2009). In the following year, 1957, an occupational therapy programme was implemented in São Paulo, initially leading to a technical qualification (Melo 2015). In the 1960s, foreign professionals established occupational therapy training in other Brazilian states.

During the period of military dictatorship, the Brazilian Centre for Health Studies, founded in 1976, became a space for discussing issues, experiences, and criticisms, aimed at the democratisation of health and society (Marques 2020). These courses were considered to be vocational courses but, in 1969, they were legally recognised as undergraduate programmes (Drummond and Cruz 2018).

From the account given here, we can see that the history of occupational therapy in Brazil is marked by strong opposition to the government, which gave the profession a solid foundation in social and political criticism.

Social activism in Brazilian occupational therapy

In the context of a military dictatorship and concomitant struggles for social rights and more humanitarian conditions in the face of massive inequality, occupational therapists in Brazil considered that their practice should encompass political action, in dialogue with problems related to or centred on the social aspects of illness and disability, such as social stigma of people with mental and disability issues, poverty and human rights. This resulted in a technical-political professional profile, not only centred on individual and group occupational therapy care but guided by the articulation of social movements that aimed to address inequality problems (Barreiro et al. 2020).

Occupational therapists in Brazil wanted to develop a professional practice that aimed to increase social participation and create a more equal society (Marcolino et al. 2020; Cardinalli and Silva 2021). Practitioners and researchers studied the works of Brazilian and European authors on topics such as pedagogy, psychoanalysis and political philosophy, such as Gilberto Freire, Paulo Freire, Sérgio Buarque de Holanda, Freud, Marx, Gramsci and Basaglia, to gain a wide understanding of social phenomena (Cardinalli 2016). Scholars and practitioners employed strong criticism to ensure that training and practice were not based on an exclusively medical and rehabilitative paradigm, and they initiated movements to direct the profession towards establishing more significant foundations for practice (Benetton 2005).

Theoretical and methodological approaches were developed within universities (Cardinalli 2016) using a materialist-historical critical perspective. These approaches include *Social Occupational Therapy* (Lopes and Malfitano 2016; 2020) and *Critical Occupational Therapy* (Galheigo 2012), both of which see occupational therapists as agents of social transformation (Barreiro et al. 2020). Outside the universities, new approaches to practice were built through study groups and clinical supervision, in a process that sought to respond to the challenges of practice, especially the daily demands experienced by professionals and clients (Lima, Pastore and Okuma 2011; Cardinalli 2016). One of these approaches is the *Dynamic Occupational Therapy Method* (DOTM), developed by Jo Benetton (Box 8.5).

Box 8.5   The Dynamic Occupational Therapy Method

Jo Benetton, the author of the DOTM, graduated in occupational therapy in 1970. At that time, students were taught to prescribe activities, for example, for people with schizophrenia or with amputations. Benetton recognised that the logic of cause and effect was missing from this level of practice, leading her to undertake a deeper study of occupational therapy. Working independently, she developed an epistemology that makes practice an object of study, which she called the *Theory of Technique*. This epistemology supported the development of theoretical and methodological understandings of occupational therapy practice that consider the dynamism and complexity of the domain of concern of the profession (Benetton 2005; Marcolino et al. 2020).

The objective of interventions based on the DOTM is to expand healthy spaces in everyday life, by enabling experiences that increase well-being and that gradually increase participation and social inclusion (Mello, Dituri and Marcolino 2020). The practitioner begins by carrying out a descriptive-analytical situational diagnostic, to reach an understanding of needs and desires, including the relevant aspects of the person's life situation, both at the micro- and macro-levels. This understanding is constructed from information that is produced and mapped in varied ways, including what the person says about him/herself and the people he/she lives with; what these people say and think about the person; the views of relevant others, including other professionals or the team; observations of what the person does; how the person talks about what she/he does, and any diagnoses (Marcolino et al. 2020; Mello, Dituri and Marcolino 2020).

Following the situational diagnostic, a triadic relationship is formed through the dynamic interactions of the occupational therapist, the person and their joint activities (Marcolino and Fantinatti 2014). Doing activities becomes a space of learning, acquisition and subjectivity, in which the person is free to make choices, build, destroy and express their emotions, desires and expectations, increasing awareness of their way of being, doing and relating. The therapeutic process includes ongoing dialogue between the occupational therapist and the person about their activities, through which they can analyse their experiences to find meaning in them (Benetton 1994: 100).

Many occupational therapists in Brazil are deeply engaged in the struggle for universal access to rights, given the numerous violations of human rights faced by the population. This is especially relevant when added to the multiple intersectionalities (race, social class, gender, geopolitical region) present in a country with great inequality. However, the aim to expand people's participation in social life through relational and creative processes creates a constant contradiction in occupational therapy (Tedesco and Maximino 2016). While social transformation is desired, and occupational therapists seek to contribute to such transformation, they also feel that their role is to help people participate in society as it is, in the expectation that this process will itself contribute to and be part of the desired social transformation (Benetton 2010).

This section used the example of occupational therapy in Brazil to show how practices change over time, in response to other, related practices. Occupational therapy in Brazil has developed into a practice entity with a distinctive character, as practitioners and scholars responded to, embraced or opposed the political and social changes taking place in their country during the second half of the 20th century.

The next section considers how these macro-level issues play out at the micro-level, in the daily performance of occupational therapy, through three case studies.

Micro-level influences on change

In this section, three case studies are used to illustrate how occupational therapy supports the change process for clients. All three cases came from mental health services in the city of São Paulo, Brazil. In each case, a Brazilian occupational therapy theory was used to support the occupational therapist's clinical reasoning: the DOTM. This theory, which is outlined in Box 8.5, was developed within and for the local context by a Brazilian occupational therapist (Benetton 1994).

These cases are complex, and the therapists had to take into account multiple issues, including but not limited to ethics; citizenship; the rights of children and adolescents; social roles; psychiatric services; social vulnerability; psychological distress; psychoactive substance use; diagnoses; abandonment, neglect and violence; the COVID-19 pandemic, and the political context. All these factors are integrated into the therapist's reasoning, using the DOTM (Arrigoni 2012).

Case study 1: A person-centred process in occupational therapy, by Rafaela Arrigoni

Eduardo, a teenager, was referred to occupational therapy at a Child and Youth Psychosocial Centre (CAPSij). I met him in the waiting room, where he sat swinging his legs, looking lost. Emaciated, Eduardo wore a woollen cap, a coat and torn sneakers. He did not make eye contact. He accompanied me to my room with his head down and hands clasped behind his back; behaviour that I associated with children who have passed through Fundação Casa.[1]

Eduardo told me he had been left in an orphanage by his parents. At the age of eight, he went to live on the streets, where he began to hear voices. He told me that he does not like enclosed places and feels free on the streets. Recently, he had started to hear the voices more often. They now told him to do things he did not want to do, such as to hurt himself and other people.

I asked Eduardo what activities he did on the streets and what had changed when the voices became more intrusive. Eduardo said that he lived on the streets 'in a good way': waking up, finding somewhere to take a shower, eating and walking. Some time ago, he started using marijuana, then cocaine and now crack cocaine. Whereas using drugs used to give him relief, now he felt despair as if his peace of mind had been stolen. He told me that writing helped him to calm down and made his thoughts more organised.

I discussed Eduardo's case with the mental health team and with professionals from other services who knew him. The preliminary medical diagnostic was a psychotic breakdown due to psychoactive substance use. However, for me, this diagnostic did not encompass the complexity reported in Eduardo's narrative. My first situational diagnostic took account of Eduardo's suffering, demonstrated through his physical posture of someone who has conflicted with the law and removed from social life. His story reflected abandonment by his parents and by the orphanage. He talked about having had a full everyday life on the streets, carrying out activities 'in a good way' until something fell apart.

In our first session, I suggested that Eduardo write down what he was thinking and feeling; my goal was to initiate the first movements of a triadic relationship. Eduardo became excited and wanted to construct a book. He chose the materials without difficulty, taking sheets of paper, folding them, punching holes, tying the book together with ribbon and writing on the cover *Book of Thoughts*. He asked to take the book with him for writing at other times, although he only read it with me.

Eduardo attended occupational therapy sessions regularly, always with the book in his pocket. When he arrived in an agitated state, he used to say that his headaches would go away when he had company for lunch, playing, talking or walking. I associated this request with his narrative of abandonment and decided to be available, whenever possible, to keep him company in these activities.

The mental health team considered Eduardo's best housing option to be a shelter, away from the dangers of the street, where his medication could be supervised. After discussing this with me, Eduardo agreed to go to the shelter.[2] However, he left after one night because he could not tolerate the lack of freedom. Following lengthy negotiations with me, he agreed to return to the shelter. Throughout this time, he remained assiduous in complying with drug treatment and attending occupational therapy; and there was a visible improvement in his mental state. He continued to express a wish to leave the shelter, where there were relationship problems with other teenagers and the shelter team. In one session, I saw that the *Book of Thoughts* contained letters addressed to me, in which he called for his freedom. In the last letter, he wrote that he was about to leave everything, not just the shelter. The situation seemed increasingly risky.

I asked myself what the most ethical action would be: listening to him and legitimising his desire or focussing on the rights set out in the *Statute of the Child and Adolescent*[3] (Brazil 1990), which was intended to guarantee freedom, respect and dignity for the developing young person. Reflecting on the contradictions within this document, the team decided it would be appropriate for Eduardo to leave the shelter. We looked around for a more suitable institution. Not all shelters had the structure to meet mental healthcare needs so Eduardo would need to spend the day at a CAPSij, only sleeping at the shelter. Transportation was difficult and the institution was not always sensitive to a request that seemed superficial in comparison with the complex needs of the children and adolescents under their care.

With Eduardo's full participation, the social worker and I advocated for him in the Guardianship Council and the Children's Court but, in the middle of this process, he ran away from the shelter and returned to live on the streets. He continued to participate in treatment at CAPSij, and in the occupational therapy sessions, but his psychiatric condition worsened. He reported suicidal ideation and asked to return to the shelter.

We found him a welcoming space in a new shelter, where he resumed psychiatric treatment. However, his other activities at CAPSij were interrupted and we had difficulty contacting him. When I called the shelter, he was never available, due to routine activities. I emphasised to shelter staff the importance of him continuing treatment and planned for him to be followed up at a primary health service close to the shelter.

Eduardo wanted to return to the CAPSij and was able to participate in a party at the centre. When I met him there, I explained how I had continued trying to help him when we were physically separated. After the party, we went to my room, and he gave me another letter. He said that the letters and the *Book of Thoughts* helped him to know that I was always there for him and would not abandon him.

Eventually, Eduardo chose to continue living on the streets, which he saw as his natural home. He received his medication monthly and we maintained communication through the pharmacy team. The last time I met him, he was clean and looked well-fed; his hands were at his sides and his legs were still. When he saw me, he smiled, looked into my eyes, gave me a big hug and said he missed me. Eduardo said he no longer needed drugs because living on the streets was now a choice and he was working as a bricklayer's helper.

I felt happy that Eduardo could see more choices in his life but, at the same time, I wanted him to attend school, live in a house and be protected from the dangers of the streets. However, I took the perspective that the therapist must silence her own desires and anxieties to allow the person to be, do and relate in their own way in their social life (Benetton 1994; Mello, Dituri and Marcolino 2020).

How change occurred in this situation?

At the beginning of Eduardo's story, he was living on the streets, taking illegal drugs and experiencing distressing psychiatric symptoms. At the end of the story, he was still living on the streets but had given up illegal drugs, was taking psychiatric medication and had found a job. Many of the material elements of Eduardo's life remained the same but, through the process of therapy, he developed new competences (making trusting relationships, building confidence, taking care of his physical and mental health) and, crucially, changed the meaning of his life on the street from a negative consequence of being abandoned to a freely chosen lifestyle.

One of the key features of Eduardo's therapy was that engagement in new activities allowed him to transfer the meaning that drug-taking had in his life (relief from distress) to other activities, including writing and talking. Another key feature of therapy was the strong, trusting relationship he formed with the occupational therapist, through the interactions of the triadic relationship (Box 8.5). This took time and progress was not straightforward; Eduardo made several attempts and failures before he could trust that he would not be abandoned again.

The occupational therapist acknowledged that she would have liked Eduardo to make more radical changes to the material elements of his life so that he would be safe, but she accepted that he was making an autonomous choice about how he lived.

Case study 2: The change process, by Ana Paula Briguet

This case study was written when I worked at a Psychosocial Care Centre for Alcohol and Other Drugs (CAPSad). This Centre offered individual care (psychiatric, occupational therapy, psychotherapy and social service) and group care (welcoming group, family group, relapse prevention group, group assemblies, outings, life project group and income generation). There was a daily reflection group, in which I participated twice a week as a co-therapist, where participants could talk about issues emerging from the treatment process, and a twice-weekly occupational therapy group that I coordinated. In the occupational therapy group, I offered participants opportunities to experiment with doing various activities that would broaden their experience and allow them to find other meanings, pleasures and goals beyond those exclusively related to drug use, which dominated their everyday lives.

In the reflection group one morning, Antonio, a 28-year-old man from Maranhão, in the northeast region of Brazil, sat in a corner of the room. He spoke little but some of his words referred to the difficulty of stopping using drugs (he had been using marijuana and crack cocaine for 13 years). He talked about the sensations provoked by drugs, saying he wanted to stop but did not want to give up the pleasure they brought.

After this session, Antonio arrived at the occupational therapy group with a restless gaze that passed quickly across the materials available. He sat upright, constantly moving his feet and hands. 'Do you think I can do something like that?' he asked, referring to the paintings on the wall. He picked up materials agitatedly as if he urgently needed something to do. I tried to reduce his restless movements by asking him to sit down and tell me what he liked to do; what were the interests that bound him to life? Antonio showed me a photograph of his one-year-old son and spoke of the two children he left in Maranhão, in the care of his grandmother. He remembered his enchantment with a travelling circus that used to come to town when he was a child. Antonio then said that he would like to paint a portrait of his son. He quickly mixed paints and painted. Even though the painting was still wet when the group ended, he took it away with him.

In another session, when people were looking at art books, Antonio said he would like to paint again. He began to leaf quickly through the books. I talked with him calmly, drawing his attention to the colours and shapes in the books, trying to slow his agitated movements. He noticed some boat shapes and chose to paint them, but said he was too anxious. This time, he allowed me to show him the range of materials and possibilities available. He began to ask for my help and opinion, which took us into the initial movements of the triadic relationship.

My first situational diagnostic, derived from these observations, included (1) the centrality of drug use in his life and how it gave him the pleasure he was not willing to forego; (2) the fast pace of his movements and activities and (3) his openness to talking about himself and to learning new things (away from drug use). I could see he was very emotional, connected to the land where he was born and to his own history. The triadic relationship was easily set up, after Antonio's initial refusal to allow my participation in the first painting, and it became possible to establish new movements as I called his attention to the activities.

After attending several group sessions, Antonio asked for individual sessions with me. The team agreed to his request because he showed emotional investment in the occupational therapy group, opening new possibilities for pleasurable experimentation in the triadic relationship, unrelated to activities connected with drug use. We arranged to have weekly individual sessions, in addition to group sessions. To enrich Antonio's learning and encourage him to take longer over each painting, I suggested he make a sketch on paper first. He drew the outline of a face with a gaping mouth and two hollow eyes, which was given a startled look by the twitching lines of the eyebrows. The drawing resembled a frown or a scowl. In another session, Antonio transferred this drawing to a canvas and began to paint more slowly, with attention to detail. This was the first activity he did not finish in one session.

During these activities, Antonio told me stories from his life, always with great emotion. He said he had worked with his father since he was little, learning to sell, trade and even deceive people. Sometimes, he became confused about what was real and what was false, often saying that his life was a farce. However, his deep involvement in painting highlighted that he was engaged in doing activities and in giving them narrative and emotional meanings. He allowed himself to learn with me, appreciate his own work and find a new, calm rhythm of working. At this time, Antonio stopped using crack but continued to use marijuana. It became increasingly evident that he was feeling threatened and persecuted. He no longer left his house alone and his wife accompanied him to the CAPSad.

After some months, Antonio moved to another city. For almost two years, there was no news of him; then he returned to the CAPSad. He had started using crack again and looked physically and emotionally fragile. A new agreement was negotiated, allowing him to attend the Centre in a way that suited him, step-by-step and to choose the activities that had the most meaning for him.

Antonio returned to our individual sessions, where he was surprised to find that his paintings had been saved. He chose a new canvas, looked carefully at it, selected the colours he was going to use and mixed the paints. He did a free painting but, at the end, saw the shape of a cat in it. He said he had had a cat in Maranhão but his mother, in one of her violent fits, had thrown it at the wall so it died.

In the next session, Antonio spontaneously chose to make a clay model of a well. While doing this, he started to cry and recounted a memory of his mother taking him to a well, holding him upside down by his legs and threatening to drop him into the dark hole. I commented how difficult this situation must have been, as he was just a child. He continued to cry: 'my mother used to beat me a lot, she would hurt me and then she would take care of me by making compresses with salt water'. After a few moments, Antonio began to cry more intensely, saying: 'sometimes we want to run away. That's what I've done my whole life; I run away from suffering, from pain'.

After this episode, Antonio began to change and realise new projects. He had not used crack for about seven months and decided to stop using marijuana. He separated from his wife, choosing to live alone for the first time. He resumed his school studies and started a theatre course. After going to the theatre for the first time, he drew the drama and comedy masks during an occupational therapy session. For Antonio, the theatre became an exciting space that offered possibilities of encounters with books, characters, people, the body and make-up. Little by little, these experiences became pleasurable for him, he said: 'Theatre gives me pleasure, as do drugs'.

Remembering his childhood experience of the circus, Antonio began to think about working as a clown at children's parties. With the support of the team, he was able to turn this desire into a work project. He began with the creation of the clown: the name, the costume, the style, the make-up, the way he would move and act and how to publicise himself. The clown's clothes were made in occupational therapy sessions; Antonio commented: 'No one has ever helped me or put so much faith in me like this'. He started to do some work as a clown, entertaining children's parties and performing in stores. At the end of the first year, he attended the Centre party as a clown.

How change occurred in this situation

When Antonio started attending occupational therapy, he had a history of ill-treatment as a child, leaving his own children behind when he moved to São Paulo and taking psychoactive drugs. He was experiencing physical and psychiatric symptoms related to both his life experiences and his drug use.

Change began for Antonio when he engaged with painting during occupational therapy sessions. This activity, together with gentle guidance from the occupational therapist became a vehicle through which he could explore the meaning of his early experiences of abuse and loss. The process was not a smooth one and there was a hiatus of two years, when Antonio moved away and started taking drugs again.

On his return to the CAPSad, Antonio found that his paintings had been retained in the occupational therapy department, providing material evidence of the concern staff felt for him. This discovery triggered the further exploration of his life experiences and the conflicting meanings many of them held. Eventually, Antonio was able to make decisions that affected many areas of his life, including relationships, drug use, education and work, all of which interacted with each other, accelerating the process of change. For this young man, occupational therapy was the catalyst for changing his material circumstances, competences and meanings.

Case study 3: Technological innovation, by Sonia Maria Leonardi Ferrari

During the COVID-19 pandemic of 2020, although the Brazilian government did not adopt a lockdown policy (The Lancet, 2020), many Brazilian health services followed World Health Organization (WHO) guidelines and introduced telehealth practices. This case study describes my experience as an expert occupational therapist, with 45 years of experience in mental health practice, running telehealth groups in a mental health day hospital during the pandemic. I discussed this practice in a partnership with three academics, one from Brazil and two from the United Kingdom, in a paper published in the *Brazilian Journal of Occupational Therapy* (Ferrari et al. 2022).

This mental health day hospital is a private service, funded by health insurance. It offers multidisciplinary care, strongly focused on group work, for people with intense psychological distress who are not economically vulnerable. Our face-to-face groups were interrupted on March 15, 2020, and emergency care only was maintained. The occupational therapy telehealth group started on March 23, amid many doubts: 'Would the online environment be suitable and appropriate for our clients? How would the sessions happen without the concrete elements of materials and tools? Above all, was physical presence an essential need for most of our clients? How could a caring relationship occur while they are in their homes, and we are in ours?' (Ferrari et al. 2022). Although not having answers to these questions, I relied on the robustness of the theoretical-methodological framework provided by the DOTM to venture into the online universe. I understood that, while the context of the interaction was changing, triadic relationships would occur in some form.

To begin the therapeutic process, the initial focus of group work was on teaching participants to use the online platform and generating proposals for suitable activities. The process of carrying out activities was like what happens in face-to-face groups, enabling all participants to carry out the same activity or each person to work individually within the context of the group. An occupational therapy group based on DOTM involves alternating these two group techniques: activities carried out collectively, with all participants doing the same activity, and each person doing their own activity in the group environment, (Ferrari 2015).

In a typical face-to-face meeting, these group dynamics are observed and encouraged by the therapist. In the online context, it was necessary to make room for each person to participate, considering: the material resources for carrying out activities in each one's home; the additional difficulties of learning a skill when the activity is carried out in an online group, and the needs and desires that emerged in this context. I also understood that this new setting would allow me to get to know the group participants in a new way, which would enrich my situational diagnostic with new information about the situation of each one, especially in this difficult time.

These group members have always liked playing games and this seemed like a good proposition, at first. But when we offered to play an online game, the participants did not engage because another participant offered to teach origami, which was a much more attractive and challenging activity for them. That person taught the others how to make an origami of a tsuru, a type of Japanese bird. After this, many other activities were carried out using materials that were commonly available in people's homes, like paper. Activities were also carried out through apps, such as sharing the screen with favourite songs and video clips. Other activities required specific apps that enabled visits to museum sites, travel through countries around the world, listening to the radio in real-time from other countries and making a group collage. For these activities to be possible, it was essential for me to master each activity process and to understand how apps and the online environment work.

Many aspects of online activity groups demanded particular attention and care, such as separating social issues from technological ones. Once, with all the participant windows open, a participant said that everyone was looking only at him. My attention was present all the time, trying to observe what was going on with each person, in each window. It was often important to explain how the virtual environment worked. Other unusual situations arose during sessions, precisely because of the virtual possibilities; for example, the group were able to accompany one of the participants, who had to undergo surgery, until she entered the operating room.

Asynchronous interactions, mainly the exchange of messages through a virtual communication app, made it possible both to choose activities ahead of group sessions and to provide emotional support to participants who were going through difficult times.

It was also possible, within the telehealth groups, to take care of the specific needs of each participant; for example, helping one of them to register and receive money from the government benefit scheme and assisting another to take a bath in their mother's house, where there was no privacy.

Two participants attending the telehealth occupational therapy group experienced unique outcomes. One of them, who had always been quite reserved in face-to-face social interactions, gradually managed to participate in the group, even sharing activities that were very personal to them. Another person, who was significantly affected by social isolation due to the COVID pandemic, managed to organise their care routine and expand their political and cultural interests.

This case study describes a specific population that is not economically vulnerable. The digital divide between rich and poor is a key factor when thinking about who can access care practices in telehealth. In Brazil, political issues have limited services to the population, including health, education, work and social assistance, due to a government that is strongly aligned with neoliberal practices and that disrespects humanitarian guidelines (The Lancet, 2020). There is still a long way to go for occupational therapists in developing and delivering equitable services. There are many questions to reflect on in the search for evidence to improve this exciting and innovative practice.

How change occurred in this situation

In this case study, change was imposed on mental health day services by the response of local healthcare providers to the COVID-19 pandemic. Along with other staff, the occupational therapist had to move from offering face-to-face group sessions at the day hospital to facilitating online group meetings. She acknowledged that this was only possible because clients using the service had sufficient resources of time and money to enable them to participate in an online community.

One of the first tasks of the therapist was to ensure that group members not only had the necessary material resources to participate in an online group but that they also had the competences. The therapist herself had to develop new competences in using different apps and online platforms so that she could teach and support the clients.

Once the telehealth group started, the therapist found that many of her existing therapeutic competences were still relevant, such as monitoring the responses of participants and using the DOTM to support her clinical reasoning. Nonetheless, some of these competences had to be used in new ways, for example, helping clients to learn technological skills as well as craft and social skills.

As participants adjusted their ways of working and interacting, and as they became more confident in using online platforms, they found that the meaning of the occupational therapy group had not changed, even though the material setting was entirely different.

Summary and conclusion

This chapter began with an exploration of change and how it occurs, using a practice theory perspective that sees practice in two ways: as an entity continuing through space and time, and as performances through which each performance and performer introduces changes to practice-as-an-entity. Through examples of the changing practices in community healthcare in the United Kingdom, the authors explored how connected and interdependent practices combine in different ways at different times. The second section of the chapter reviewed the influence of macro-level issues on the development and performance of occupational therapy in Brazil, to produce a development and focus that are characteristic of the national profession. The final part of the chapter used three case studies, based on a Brazilian occupational therapy theory, the DOTM, to highlight the micro-level changes that occurred during intervention. Two case studies described how change occurred for vulnerable clients during their engagement with services. A third case study described changes brought about for the attendees of a mental health day service during the COVID-19 pandemic. The changing life context of individual clients and the impact of COVID-19 on how the group could meet necessitated alterations in the occupational therapist's practice performance. Each of these three interventions was analysed from a practice theory perspective, using the elements of materials, competences and meanings to explain how the change came about.

Notes

1 The Fundação CASA is an Adolescent Socio-Educational Service Centre is a foundational autarchy (legal entity governed by public law) created by the Government of the State of São Paulo (Brazil) and linked to the Secretary of State for Justice and Defence of Citizenship. Its function is to carry out the socio-educational measures applied by the Judiciary to teenagers who committed infractions under the age of 18. At the Fundação Casa, they can serve a prison sentence up to the age of 21, as determined by the Statute of Children and Adolescents (ECA). See https://pt.wikipedia.org/wiki/Funda%C3%A7%C3%A3o_CASA

2 Institutional Shelter Services for Children and Adolescents (SAICA is the acronym in Portuguese) are arranged as protective measures for children and adolescents at personal or social risk or in conditions of abandonment. Various institutions can request places, for example, through the judicial process, by specialised referral centres in social assistance and through health institutions, such as CAPS.

3 The 1990 Statute of the Child and Adolescent/ECA (the acronym in Portuguese is for Estatuto da Criança e do Adolescente) is a Brazilian law resulting from a collaboration involving parliamentarians, government, social movements, researchers, institutions for the defence of the rights of children and adolescents and international organisations. Children and adolescents are seen as having rights; of being in a condition of development and of having absolute priority for protection. The law affirms the responsibility of the family, society and the State to guarantee conditions for the full development of this population, in addition to protecting them from all forms of discrimination, exploitation and violence (Brazil 1990).

References

Abdu, L., and Cooper, K. (2016) The implications of mobile working for health visiting practice. *Journal of Health Visiting*, 4(7): 360–364.

Arrigoni, R. (2012) Onde habitar é possível [Where it is possible to live]. *Revista CETO*, 13, 67–73. Online at https://ceto.pro.br/wp-content/uploads/2021/03/09-arrigoni-1.pdf. Accessed May 2022.

Audi, R. (1999) *The Cambridge Dictionary of Philosophy*, 2nd edition. Cambridge: Cambridge University Press.

Barreiro, R.G., Borba, P.L.O., and Malfitano, A.P.S. (2020) Revisitando o materialismo histórico em Terapia Ocupacional: O papel técnico, ético e político na contemporaneidade [Revisiting historical materialism in occupational therapy: its technical, ethical and political role in contemporary times]. *Cadernos Brasileiros de Terapia Ocupacional*, 28(4): 1311–1321. 10.4322/2526-8910.ctoRE1950

Barros, F.B.M. (2009) Fisioterapia, poliomielite e filantropia: A ABBR e a Formação do fisioterapeuta no Rio de Janeiro (1954–1965) [Physiotherapy, poliomyelitis and philanthropy: ABBR and the training of the physiotherapist in Rio de Janeiro (1954–1965)]. Doctoral thesis. Rio de Janeiro: Fundação Oswaldo Cruz, Casa de Oswaldo Cruz. Online at https://www.arca.fiocruz.br/handle/icict/6153. Accessed May 2022.

Benetton, M.J. (1994) A Terapia Ocupacional como instrumento nas ações de Saúde mental [Occupational therapy as a tool in mental health actions]. Doctoral thesis. Campinas, Brazil: Universidade de Campinas.

Benetton, M.J. (2005) Além da opinião: Uma questão de investigação para a historicização da Terapia Ocupacional [Beyond opinion: a research question for the historicization of occupational therapy]. *Revista CETO*, 9: 4–8.

Benetton, J. (2010) O encontro do sentido do Cotidiano na Terapia Ocupacional para a construção de significados [Finding the meaning of everyday life in occupational therapy for the construction of meanings]. *Revista CETO*, 12: 32–39.

Blue, S., and Spurling, N. (2017) Qualities of connective tissue in hospital life. In: A. Hui, T. Achatzki , and E. Shove (eds.) *The nexus of practices: connections, constellations, practitioners*. London: Routledge. 24–37.

Brasil (1988) Constitution of the Federative republic of Brazil. Online at https://www.constituteproject.org/constitution/Brazil_2017.pdf?lang=en. Accessed May 2022.

Brasil (2004) Saúde mental no SUS: Os centros de atenção psicossocial [Mental health in the SUS: psychosocial care centers]. Brasília-DF: Ministério da Saúde. Online at http://portal.saude.gov.br/portal/arquivos/pdf/manual_caps.pdf. Accessed May 2022.

Brasil (2013) Conheça a RAPS: Rede de atenção psicossocial [Get to know RAPS: Psychosocial Care Network]. Brasília-DF: Ministério da Saúde. Online at https://bvsms.saude.gov.br/bvs/folder/conheca_raps_rede_atencao_psicossocial.pdf. Accessed May 2022.

Brazil (1990) Brazil: Statute of the Child and Adolescent [Brazil], Law no 8.069, 13 July 1990, available at: https://www.refworld.org/docid/4c481bcf2.html [accessed 18 July 2022].

Cardinalli, I. (2016) Conhecimentos da Terapia Ocupacional no Brasil: Um estudo sobre trajetórias e produções [Knowledge of occupational therapy in Brazil: a study on trajectories and productions]. Masters dissertation. São Carlos: UFSCar. Online at https://repositorio. ufscar.br/handle/ufscar/8496. Accessed May 2022.

Cardinalli, I., and Silva, C.R. (2021) Atividades humanas na Terapia Ocupacional: Construção e compromisso [Human activities in occupational therapy: construction and commitment]. *Cadernos Brasileiros de Terapia Ocupacional*, 29: e2880. 10.1590/2526-8910.ctoAO2176

de Certeau, M. (1984). *The practice of everyday life*, trans. Steven Rendall. Berkeley: University of California Press.

Drummond, A.D., and Cruz, D.M. (2018) History of occupational therapy in Brazil: inequalities, advances, and challenges. *Annals of International Occupational Therapy*, 1(2): 103–112. 10.3928/24761222-20180409-01

Escorel, S. (1999) *Reviravolta na saúde: origem e articulação do movimento sanitário*. Brazil: FIOCRUZ. https://doi.org/10.7476/9788575413616

Ferguson, H. (2009) Driven to care: the car, automobility and social work. *Mobilities*, 4(2): 275–293.

Ferrari, M.A.C. (2013) A light at the end of the tunnel of knowledge: the arrival of occupational therapy in the city of Sao Paulo. *Cadernos de Terapia Ocupacional da UFSCar*, 21(3): 663–670. 10.4322/cto.2013.069

Ferrari, S.M.L. (2015) Grupos de Terapia Ocupacional em saúde mental: Novas reflexões [Occupational therapy groups in mental health: new reflections]. In: V.S. Maximino and F. Liberman (eds.) *Grupos e Terapia Ocupacional: Formação, pesquisa e ações*. São Paulo: Summus Editorial. 226–237.

Ferrari, S.M.L., Pywell, S.D., Costa, A.L.B.D., and Marcolino, T.Q. (2022) Occupational therapy telehealth groups in COVID-19 pandemic: perspectives from a mental health day hospital. *Cadernos Brasileiros de Terapia Ocupacional*, 30: e3019. 10.1590/2526-8910.ctoRE22 883019

Fiocruz (2015) Fundação Oswaldo Cruz, Fundação Calouste Gulbenkian. Inovações e Desafios em Desinstitucionalização e Atenção Comunitária no Brasil [Innovations and challenges in deinstitutionalization and community care in Brazil]. In: *Seminário Internacional de Saúde Mental: Documento Técnico*. Rio de Janeiro: Fundação Oswaldo Cruz (Fiocruz), Fundação Calouste Gulbenkian, Organização Mundial de Saúde (OMS), Ministério da Saúde (MS).

Galheigo, S. (2012) Perspectiva Crítica y Compleja de Terapia Ocupacional: Actividad, Cotidiano, Diversidad, Justicia social y Compromiso Ético-político [A critical and complex perspective of occupational therapy: activity, daily, diversity, social justice and ethical-political commitment]. *Revista de Terapia Ocupacional Galicia* (TOG - A Coruña), Galícia, 9: 176–187.

Greenlees, J. (2018) To care and educate: the continuity within Queen's nursing in Scotland, c. 1948–2000. *Nursing History Review*, 26(1): 97–110.

Instituto Brasileiro de Geografia e Estatística (2022). Online at https://www.ibge.gov.br. Accessed May 2022.

Jeyasingham, D. (2020) Entanglements with offices, information systems, laptops and phones: how agile working is influencing social workers' interactions with each other and with families. *Qualitative Social Work*, 19(3): 337–358.

Lima, E.M.F.A., Pastore, M.N., and Okuma, D.G. (2011) As atividades no campo da Terapia Ocupacional: Mapeamento da produção científica dos terapeutas ocupacionais Brasileiros de 1990 a 2008 [Activities in the field of occupational therapy: mapping of the scientific production of two Brazilian occupational therapists from 1990 to 2008]. *Revista de Terapia Ocupacional da Universidade de São Paulo*, 22: 68–75.

Lopes, R.E., and Malfitano, A.P.S. (2016) *Terapia Ocupacional Social: Desenhos teóricos e contornos práticos*. São Carlos: Edufscar.

Lopes, R.E., and Malfitano, A.P.S. (eds.) (2020) *Social occupational therapy: theoretical and practical designs*. Edinburgh: Elsevier Health Sciences.

Lussi, I.A.O., Ferigato, S.H., Gozzi, A.P.N.F., Fernandes, A.D.S.A., Morato, G.G., Cid, M.F.B., Marcolino, T.Q., and Matsukura, T.S. (2019). Saúde mental em pauta: Afirmação do cuidado em liberdade e resistência aos retrocessos [Mental health in guidelines: affirmation of care in freedom and resistance to setbacks]. *Cadernos Brasileiros de Terapia Ocupacional*, 27(1): 1–3. 10.4322/2526-8910.ctoED2701

Machado, C.V., and Silva, G.A.E. (2019) Political struggles for a universal health system in Brazil: successes and limits in the reduction of inequalities. *Global Health*, 15: 77. 10.1186/s12992-019-0523-5

Marcolino, T.Q., Benetton, J., Cestari, L.M.Q., Mello, A.C.C., and Araújo, A.S. (2020). Dialogues with Benetton and Latour: possibilities for an understanding of social insertion. *Cadernos Brasileiros de Terapia Ocupacional*, 28(4): 1322–1334. 10.4322/2526-8910.ctoARF2032

Marcolino, T.Q., and Fantinatti, E.N. (2014). A transformação na utilização e conceituação de atividades na obra de Jô Benetton [A transformation in the use and design of activities in the work of Jô Benetton]. *Revista De Terapia Ocupacional Da Universidade De São Paulo*, 25(2): 142–150. 10.11606/issn.2238-6149.v25i2p142-150

Marques, I.P. (2020) A saúde mental brasileira sob o olhar decolonial: Contribuições para o debate da saúde mental global a partir de uma experiência de cooperação internaCional com a Itália [Brazilian mental health from a decolonial perspective: contributions to the global mental health debate based on an experience of international cooperation with Italy]. Doctoral thesis. Universidade Federal de São Carlos, São Carlos. Online at https://repositorio.ufscar.br/handle/ufscar/12712. Accessed May 2022.

Marques, I.P., Ferigato, S.H., Minelli, M., and Marcolino, T.Q. (2020) Da produção local à cooperação Internacional em Saúde mental: Construção de redes de cuidado e aprendizagem entre Brasil e Itália [From local production to international cooperation in mental health: building care and learning networks between Brazil and Italy]. *Interface - Comunicação, Saúde, Educação*, 24. 10.1590/Interface.200241.

Mello, A.C.C., Dituri, D.R., and Marcolino, T.Q. (2020) The meaning making of what is meaningful: dialogues with Wilcock and Benetton. *Cadernos Brasileiros de Terapia Ocupacional*, 28(1): 352–373.

Melo, D.O.C.V. (2015) *Em Busca de um Ethos*: Narrativas da Fundação da Terapia Ocupacional na Cidade de São Paulo (1956–1969). Masters thesis. São Paulo: UNIFESP. Online at https://repositorio.unifesp.br/handle/11600/45786. Accessed May 2022.

Salles, M.M., Barros, S., and Matsukura, T.S. (2016) The Brazilian community mental health care services: social inclusion and psychosocial rehabilitation. *Journal of Psychosocial Rehabilitation and Mental Health*, 3: 89–94. 10.1007/s40737-016-0067-4

Schwarz, L.M., and Starling, H.M. (2018) *Brazil: a biography*. London: Penguin.

Serapioni, M. (2019) Franco Basaglia: biography of a revolutionary. *História, Ciências, Saúde-Manguinhos*, 26: 1169–1187.

Shorter Oxford English Dictionary (2002) *Shorter Oxford English Dictionary*. Oxford: Oxford University Press.

Shove, E., Pantzar, M. , and Watson, M. (2012) *The dynamics of social practice: everyday life and how it changes*. Los Angeles: Sage.

Soares, L.B.T. (1991) *Occupational therapy: logic of capital or work?* São Paulo, Brasil: Hucitec.

Tedesco, S., and Maximino, V.S. (2016) Rotina, hábitos, cotidiano: Do banal ao sutil no encantamento da vida [Routine, habits, daily life: from the banal to the subtle in the enchantment of life]. In: T.S. Matsukura and M.M. Salles (eds.) *Cotidiano, atividade humana e ocupação*: *perspectivas da terapia ocupacional no campo da saúde mental*. São Carlos: EdUFSCar. 123–146.

The Lancet (2020) COVID-19 in Brazil: "so what?" *The Lancet*, 395 (10235): 1461. 10.1016/S0140-6736(20)31095-3

UNDP (United Nations Development Programme) (2019) Human Development Report 2019: Beyond income, beyond averages, beyond today: Inequalities in human development in the 21st century. New York. https://hdr.undp.org/content/human-development-report-2019

United Nations Development Programme (2020) *Human development report 2019*. United Nations.

9 Where we want to be

Nick Pollard and Jennifer Creek

Introduction

In this chapter, we draw together some of the major themes that were explored through a practice theory lens in Chapters 1–8. These themes include the differences between occupational therapy in mainstream services and in marginal settings; the major social issues that occupational therapists are called upon to address in the 21st century, and the elements of occupational therapy as a social practice.

The first section summarises the differences between occupational therapy as a biomedical practice, operating within mainstream services, and occupational therapy as social activism. Both practices have a role in modern health and social care, and neither should be accorded higher status than the other within the profession. The second section describes some of the major social issues we face in the 21st century. Occupational therapists find that familiar ways of working are inadequate to address these issues, which are complex and challenging. Their response is to develop new theories and approaches, drawing on philosophies and epistemologies from a variety of disciplines and from cultures that have been under-represented in the profession's knowledge base. The third section outlines the elements of occupational therapy as a social practice: materials, competences, meanings and structures. A case study is used to show how these elements interact in occupational therapy practice.

Occupational therapy: Two social practices

In 2017, the American Occupational Therapy Association celebrated 100 years of the profession. In her presidential address which was published in a celebratory issue of the *American Journal of Occupational Therapy*, Amy Lamb (2017) looked back on the past and forward to a vision of the future where occupational therapy embraces in-novation and change, with a focus on high-quality services based on relevant and participatory occupation rather than mere remedial exercise. She called for therapists to look beyond insurance and reimbursement to the occupations that enrich the ex-periences of people in their daily lives and to population health issues, associated with the demographics of ageing, that enable people to retain their freedoms.

Lamb's address speaks to two practices of occupational therapy: one aligned with medical goals and processes, the other with social justice and reform. This section discusses these intertwined practices, which have been identifiable throughout the history of the profession (Mattingly and Fleming 1994; Hooper and Wood 2002).

DOI: 10.4324/9781003016755-9

Occupational therapy as a biomedical practice

Much of the practice of healthcare in western society is conceptualised as intervention; a technical process that has evolved from informal care into a complex combination of biomedical assessments and processes; involving instruments, tools, physical procedures and psychological treatments. These processes are intended to produce diagnoses, treatment plans, treatment regimes and outcomes. Occupational therapy approaches that evolved within this paradigm of intervention incorporate a range of assessment tools, procedures and methods, which the practitioner has to be trained to use. An example of one of these approaches, with a suite of tools to support it, is the Model of Human Occupation (MOHO) (Parkinson et al. 2011). One of the problems with this development is the gap between the construction of the profession as a biomedical practice and its broader understanding of activity in the context of everyday life (Bukhave and Creek 2021).

The technologies around healthcare have evolved over time to become the preserve of licensed specialists, whose knowledge of and adherence to accepted rules and processes are indicated by their possession of a professional qualification. Different authorities, such as governments and employing organisations, attempt to co-ordinate or set limits to professional practice through imposing structures and processes for education, professional recognition and standards (Weisz et al. 2007). As discussed in Chapter 1, professions seek to retain their autonomy by regulating their own business: establishing standards for procedures, processes, training and research in order to ensure approaches to practice are seen to be based on evidence.

For occupational therapy, social structures and processes define its shape as practice-as-entity; that is, as a set of materials, competences and meanings that are enacted through the practice-as-performance of professional interventions (Nicolini 2012; Shove, Pantzar and Watson 2012). Occupational therapy is thus structured as a social practice, while still having scope to develop through the further creation of materials, refinement of competences and new understanding of meanings (Nicolini 2012).

Some of the recent influences on occupational therapy as a social practice have been: the development of technology; increased standardisation of equipment, assessment tools and approaches (**materials**); the growth of specialisation throughout the 20th century, and clarification of the **competences** required for various clinical practices. Looking back to the emergence of key occupational therapy approaches, such as the MOHO and the Canadian Model of Occupational Performance, both of which were developed in the latter part of the 20th century and both of which have complex assessment batteries and instruments, it is possible to see these as representing technological apparatus for the management of needs (**meanings**) in the people with whom occupational therapists work.

The political philosopher, Gramsci (1971), was particularly interested in the emergence of technological roles and how the professionals who occupy them have a special place in the hegemonic structures of Western society. The layer of specialists that includes police, teachers and government administrators, as well as those in the clinical professions and social work, effectively control access to the resources of the hegemony for alleviating illness and poverty or for addressing such needs as education and basic protection under the law. These specialists are interposed as a barrier to preserve the interests of the hegemony from those lower in the hierarchical structure of social class. Through welfare measures eked out by administrators and immediate needs being met by professionals, matters are prevented from coalescing into a more organised expression of dissatisfaction and evolving into a threat to the status quo.

Specialists who work in systems where resources are not provided in ways that meet the health needs of clients may find that the goals and rules of the organisation conflict with their professional values (Townsend 1993, 1998). For occupational therapy, this raises significant issues of justice when, as a result of those systems, people are unable to access what they need to support everyday life (Townsend and Marval 2013). Regulation and standardisation are necessary requirements for setting economically sustainable limits to services, promoting fairness and equity and ensuring that legal requirements are met. However, they can also put professionals in awkward positions when the meaning of their practice is challenged because budget constraints prevent them from meeting client needs that have been competently assessed.

Occupational therapy and social reform

Lamb's (2017) presidential address echoes themes that recur throughout the histories of the occupational therapy profession. While Lamb drew on the stories of pioneering American occupational therapists, such as Eleanor Clarke Slagle, Wilma West and Elnora Gilfoyle, Wilcock (2001a) traced similar veins in her history of occupational therapy in the United Kingdom, with its roots in the social reformism of Octavia Hill and the Christian socialism of the late 19th century, in the face of extreme poverty with its consequent poor health and life quality.

A recognition of urgency for social change has always been a powerful motivator within the profession. As we saw in Chapters 5 and 8, Latin American accounts of occupational therapy show how the profession originated with trade missions and other, softer political influences supporting global power blocks (Monzeli, Morrison and Lopes 2019); or has sometimes been endorsed through dictatorial regimes (Lopes and Malfitano 2020). As the profession evolved, practitioners in South America similarly engaged with the urgency of social transformation, developing practices directed at countering the effects of poverty and vulnerability amongst populations at the extremes of differences in health outcomes.

This recurring impulse for reform, for occupational therapy to influence life quality through enabling healthy participation in a broad and complex range of activities, is identified in Wilcock's (2001b) first part of the history of occupational therapy in the United Kingdom. Several of the contributing authors offered anecdotal, antecedent examples from medieval and ancient history, in which the value of an enabling concern with participation in occupation was linked to better health. To date, a direct link has not been identified between these ancient precursors and the profession of occupational therapy. Tracing the evolution of a practice is difficult and leads the researcher to diverse sources and origins (Shove, Pantzar and Watson 2012), even within a profession as recent as occupational therapy.

The origins of occupational therapy as a social practice should not be narrowly centred on the relationship between the idea of occupation and the concept of therapy. A broader conceptualisation of occupation, based in an understanding of doing, being, becoming and belonging (Wilcock 1998; Hitch, Pépin and Stagnitti 2014) as the participative components of social practices (Nicolini 2012), suggests something more than the application of a technology of intervention in clinical contexts. Participation includes interaction, collaboration, co-production and collective actions, which may lead to multiple outcomes since they draw on the influences, needs and capacities of whoever is involved. Daily life occupations cannot be performed in a closed laboratory but depend upon contextual relations, as will be discussed in relation to the ecology of human performance (Dunn 2017) and other occupational therapy approaches.

Occupational therapy is concerned with the performance of social practices (Bukhave and Creek 2021), a professional purpose that should be an insurance against obsolescence and a basis for productive work with communities and individuals. However, the profession is at a critical point in considering how its future practice will look. Occupational therapists have long had an interest in forms of community development and, more recently, have begun to articulate this as social transformation (van Bruggen et al. 2020). The next section considers some of the social issues that fall within the remit of occupational therapy.

Social issues of the 21st century

Around the world, poverty and vulnerability have a complex relationship with health (Wilkinson and Pickett 2010). Lack of access to education, good food, good housing, safe and well-balanced work opportunities, free time, social activities and the maintenance of family and friendships impacts physical and mental health in a trajectory that acquires greater complexity through the life course, as health conditions accumulate and exert a greater effect. Of course, these concerns are impacted by environmental conditions, infrastructure and the availability of good and stable government, for example, but Wilkinson and Pickett (2010) point out that the key issue is that of how people experience their daily lives in relation to others in the same society.

Socio-cultural issues of access have a material impact on activities of daily living in ways that are detrimental to health over time, enacted through a pyramid of perceived status. Some jobs have a higher social status than others, while people who are out of work are generally accorded the lowest status unless they are wealthy. The privileges of material access enable people at upper levels of the pyramid to regard those at lower tiers as lacking competence. Punitive benefit systems, structural poverty and inequality create a diminishing scale of resources.

In this section, we examine three of the major social issues with which occupational therapy is grappling: the digital world, development needs and complexity.

The digital world

The end of the 20th and beginning of the 21st centuries were characterised by the incorporation of information technology and systems into many everyday social practices, such as communication and education. Making strategic use of technology has the potential to open up possibilities for people to adjust to their circumstances and sustain an acceptable standard of living (Graham 2017). However, technology can also act as an agent of marginalisation, as described in the example in Chapter 6 (Box 6.6).

One of the problems the recent development of information technology presents for people with limited incomes, particularly within what has been called the 'tethered economy' (Hoofnagle, Kesari and Perzanowski 2019: 783), is that the value derived from equipment is often not worth the financial investment required. Consumer choices are restricted or enforced through contracts with service providers and, in rural areas, accessibility might be limited and networks are sometimes unreliable. Most equipment is expensive to repair and modern technology often has a built-in short life expectancy. Software and conditions of usage may be tied into contracts, making it difficult for the purchaser to bypass them and use the equipment with a cheaper service provider. In poorer societies, people have to be conservative about purchasing expensive items, such as cars, which have built-in deterioration. One tactic is to look for fewer gimmicks to go wrong and for equipment that can be readily serviced (Çaya 2016).

It has been noted that the position of people without jobs, and those on low incomes, will worsen as society becomes more commodified and as access to resources is increasingly based on spending power (Delhey, Schneickert and Steckermeier 2017). This trajectory is about both the structure of health and social care systems as commodities and also about how other services interact with them. Access to services and other resources, such as information, increasingly relies on the use of the internet and mobile phones; for example, call systems and telehealth systems. Divergences in access to digital technologies, and hence to healthcare, are likely to become life and death matters, if they have not already done so (Lythreatis, Singh and El-Kassar 2021).

A digital divide is emerging between those who have access to online systems and those who do not have the necessary material resources, educational level, confidence or supportive culture that promotes agile thinking. Without the necessary facilities, people may find they are isolated and unable to obtain essential treatments or services. A major barrier to access comes from living in an area with poor connectivity, without infrastructure or lacking the capacity to invest in communication and intelligent systems (Thomas et al. 2018; Drury and Lazuardi 2021). The impact of such differences became rapidly apparent during the COVID-19 pandemic (Drury and Lazuardi 2021; Lythreatis, Singh and El-Kassar 2021; Chadwick et al. 2022).

Within the occupational therapy literature, many positives have been identified as coming with digital healthcare (e.g., Nobakht et al. 2017; Ninnis et al. 2019). However, there are also disadvantages, such as digital marginalisation (Box 9.1) or even digital erasure, where a person without a device is invisible to the systems that other people can use. For example, many systems and services require users to possess a mobile phone or an email account, through which they can be contacted. This measure means that in order to access one service a person must have enough income to own such devices and pay for other services connected with them, as well as being able to afford the rent for a place to live so as to have an address.

Box 9.1   Digital marginalisation

During the COVID-19 pandemic, some people experienced multiple risks while shopping for food: steering their shopping trolley through a supermarket of potentially contaminated items; pushing a trolley that may not have been adequately cleaned; paying cash at the checkout, and encountering potentially infectious people. Retail workers were identified as a group who were more exposed to infection and risk of mortality through contact with the public. People in lower-income and black and ethnic minority groups generally had higher rates of infection because of the types of work available to them, needing to use supermarkets to buy essentials, especially as flexible opening times allowed them access around their shift hours. Others, with more access to digital skills and resources, could more easily isolate themselves from others who may expose them to infection risk; for example, they could shop for groceries online and have them delivered. Such inequalities added significantly to the risks faced by some people but not by other, more advantaged groups (Public Health England 2020; Litchfield, Shukla and Greenfield 2021)

One consequence of rapid technological development is that those who are impoverished, disabled or excluded, whether through cultural, economic or geopolitical status, become increasingly marginalised. Digital developments may both enhance and exacerbate issues of access, affecting different groups in diverse ways according to their resources and capacities. Social practices may be determined not by contracts and restricted usage of equipment but also by whether a person has access to facilities at all (Hoofnagle, Kesari and Perzanowski 2019; Lythreatis, Singh and El-Kassar 2021).

Digitalisation can also pose problems for collaboration when people are unable to share the same online platform. This may be because they cannot afford or do not have access to compatible equipment, they are unable to use the equipment or they lack particular software through which information is shared (Greer et al. 2019). While digital technologies can be enabling for some people, they have the effect of excluding others; for example, those who have to use a shared or borrowed phone or laptop, or who cannot download or use software that is common to other people with whom they are collaborating. Some systems contain barriers that exclude people; for example, through gate-keeping measures or because people have to depend on others to help them access online facilities, such as carers (Chadwick et al. 2022). As socioeconomic divisions widen, there is increasing evidence to suggest that barriers associated with the digital divide are also growing (Thomas et al. 2018; Greer et al. 2019; Drury and Lazuardi 2021; Lythreatis, Singh and El-Kassar 2021).

Development needs

In this chapter, as in earlier chapters of the book, we have acknowledged that increasing economic inequality across the world is leading to growing health inequality. Not only are more people being deprived of the resources they need to support health and well-being but access to healthcare is also becoming more difficult. In response to what Oxfam has called 'the global inequality crisis', occupational therapists are exploring new approaches to providing accessible, sustainable services for communities. Many of these approaches draw on development theory rather than biomedical theory.

Some occupational therapy theories have been organised into participative and collaborative models, such as the ecology of human performance (Dunn, Brown and McGuigan 1994; Dunn 2017). Such models lead to occupation-based ways of working that focus on vulnerabilities, diversities or community development needs; for example, social occupational therapy (Lopes and Malfitano 2020), the occupation-based community development framework (Galvaan and Peters 2014) and the earlier Australian Occupational Performance Model (AOPM) (Chapparo and Ranka 1997).

These models and approaches can be considered as ways in which the profession has sought to engage in the real world of doing, being, becoming and belonging (Bukhave and Creek 2021). The ecology of human performance model, for example, identifies context as a factor in task performance, breaking it down into specific barriers for which solutions can be found by working with all the people around an individual (Dunn 2017). These approaches also produce collaborative ways of leading, through which the profession can contribute to health structures and organisations (Geilinger et al. 2016). Social occupational therapy, the occupation-based community development framework and the AOPM all emphasise working with communities rather than working for or doing things to people. They are about working together for shared outcomes, determined by community needs.

Occupational therapists working outside mainstream health and social care settings often have to make use of the resources available to them in the environment (see Chapter 7), rather than relying on specialist medical equipment. They need to be resourceful and flexible in responding to complex needs in underdeveloped settings (Creek and Cook 2017). This is illustrated by the examples in Box 9.2.

Box 9.2 Improvisation

One of the consequences of the COVID-19 pandemic was that therapists had to improvise or adapt rapidly to sustain services (e.g., see Chapter 8). New technologies were adopted to manage interventions, as patients were often in isolation, and therapists had to negotiate new ways of working with them, using whatever might be available in their domestic environments. This change in occupational therapy practice is based in a skill and social practice of improvisation, which has consistently been valued in the history of the profession (Wilcock 2001a) and is key to sustaining practice (Shove, Pantzar and Watson 2012). In the early days, occupational therapy interventions were often based on the adoption of whatever means were available; a large part of Macdonald's (1961) account of setting up a training programme in Argentina, explored in Chapter 5, concerns exactly this process. A survey carried out by Hoel and colleagues (2021) during the pandemic gives many recent examples of adapting therapeutic approaches and materials.

In Chapter 5, we explored some aspects of sustainable practice, which might contribute to action for degrowth. These can be developed by individual practitioners (Ikiugu 2008) and the profession (World Federation of Occupational Therapists 2018) as social practices oriented to the wider global community. Social practice theory admits the potential of grass-roots practices to develop and influence meso- or macro-level practice through innovation (Shove, Pantzar and Watson 2012).

Complexity

Occupational therapy is a profession that works with the complexity of doing, being, becoming and belonging, in a society of exponential growth and complicated entanglements. We have explored some of the complications that arise through digital technology solutions to care needs. There is also a growing concern about the complex connections between the sustainability of a living planet and health in humans, animals, plants and the wider economy, as represented in the United Nations 2030 development goals (Brymer, Freeman, and Richardson 2019; Lueddeke et al. 2017; UN n.d.).

In the clinical sciences, there is a pervasive tendency to reduce complexity to a process, rather than trying to comprehend the wider contexts that are part of all social practices. Such reductionism can lead to occupation being taken for granted and mistaken as everyday and simple (Pentland, 2021). Lamb (2017) identified occupation as an underpinning concept for the occupational therapy profession and a potential source of power. Perhaps this is so but Pentland (2021) referred to Greenhalgh and Papoutsi's (2018) earlier commentary on the need, within the medical sciences, for new paradigms that address complexity in terms of social, economic, political, cultural and environmental factors.

From an occupational therapy perspective, one of the problems of trying to work with complexity concerns the occupational dimension of human inter-relationships with the rest of humanity, and with nature itself, through participative doing (Mourão et al. 2022). The curriculum of the first occupational therapy training programmes included traditional activities, such as country dancing, as well as crafts, such as weaving and basket making. Early interventions included rural activities, such as gardening and livestock management (Wilcock 2001a), with some psychiatric hospitals including farms and orchards where patients were expected to work. A recent resurgence of interest in gardening and horticulture is highlighting these activities as a means of developing various technical skills, alongside other communal forms of shared and accessible doing (Mourão et al. 2022).

In an attempt to theorise the complexity of establishing and maintaining communal relationships through doing, occupational therapists have sought explanations that can be incorporated into the knowledge base of the profession. A number of these are collective or unifying ideas that revolve around forms of collaboration. One such concept is *ubuntu* (Box 9.3), a term that has been popular in professional education, social care and health terminologies in South Africa since majority rule, from which time it became one of the principles for rebuilding a diverse, post-apartheid society.

Box 9.3   Ubuntu

Ubuntu is a concept that has many parallels across sub-Saharan Africa. While the concept is often used when referring to mutual aid, there are depths that require a firm grounding in the various interpretations of ubuntu before trying to apply them to practice (van Breda 2019). Ubuntu addresses many aspects of the ways in which people can be mindful of each other in relation to their participation in occupation and social practices. The collective concept in occupational therapy's participatory principle is echoed in the Zulu maxim 'umuntu ngumunthu ngabantu': 'a person is a person through persons' (Joubert 2009: 1). This saying implies that human meaning comes out of what people do together. In other words, a person is an individual because of their interconnection with a group in the performance of social practices. It is not only what we do together as human beings that makes participation possible but also our differences and our autonomy.

Ubuntu challenges aspects of inequality; for example, extreme differences in health outcomes, such as incidence of disease or divergences in life expectancy within a community. The ubuntu principle that 'whatever one does to another, he or she does it to himself or herself' (Chuwa 2014: 10) means that people cannot be unfairly exploited by others because we are all interdependent; to treat a person in an inhuman way is to diminish one's own qualities as a human. Ubuntu can be a useful perspective from which to examine justice in social practices throughout the world, and perhaps to frame solutions to problems, since its implications relate to the entirety of social practices.

Caution must be exercised in using collective ideas with insufficient understanding (Walton 2018). The concept of ubuntu has been exploited to endorse ideologies such as neoliberal policy values, which are far from collective in their endorsement of competition and production of inequality. Such misuse of ubuntu principles sometimes results in the popular rejection of its potentially inclusive values rather than a critical consideration of their relevance for good practice (McDonald 2010; Fung 2015). When applying collective principles such as ubuntu to occupational therapy practice, significant challenges arise from the counter-principles of the dominant ideology of many of the settings where occupational therapists work. These challenges have to be critically understood and addressed in creating a strategic, participative path to change.

One of the tasks for health researchers, particularly those concerned with health promotion or disease prevention, is to identify how the relationship between human and planetary health works (Brymer, Freeman and Richardson 2019). This is an objective that could underpin such projects as the UK's *NHS long term plan* (2019). This plan seeks to address the relationship between demographic changes and the increasing complexity of comorbidities, through providing community-based services that involve multiple agencies. Such approaches are grounded in a stronger sense of reality than the clinical perspective alone but they are likely to be multifactorial and complex, requiring a participatory form of citizen engagement if they are to be effected sustainably (Fung 2015; Pollard et al. 2020).

This section reviewed some of the major social issues that provide the context for occupational therapy practice. The next section identifies some additional elements of occupational therapy as a social practice.

Elements of occupational therapy as a social practice

In this section, we review the elements that make up occupational therapy as a social practice. These elements are grouped under four headings: materials, competences, meanings and structures, with a discussion of the contributions of the previous chapters to these themes. A case study follows, illustrating one way in which one occupational therapist is combining these elements in a successful practice.

Materials

Many of the occupational therapy work settings described in this book are not traditional hospital environments but marginal spaces, such as refugee camps and community centres. These settings incorporate very different materials and other resources from those found in healthcare organisations and, consequently, the practices of occupational therapists working in them develop differently, in relation to the material environment.

Shove and colleagues (2012) described materials as 'the hardware of everyday life' (p. 10); which includes 'objects, infrastructures, tools [...] and the body itself' (p. 23). All social practices are tied to the arrangement of artefacts, materials and technologies (Schatzki 2010) in the environment, because material things are an essential element of a social practice. For example, cooking requires some form of ingredients, utensils, tools and heat source as essential elements of performance. Furthermore, the way the practice is performed is shaped by what is available for use in the environment. Materials become resources when they are utilised in the performance of practices.

Chapter 7 discussed the people and things that constitute resources for occupational therapy practice: personal capabilities, material resources, space-time and human resources. Macro-level factors, including economics and politics, influence the availability of material resources in diverse settings, and how they can be used. Case studies from marginal settings were used to illustrate the significance of resourcefulness as a professional attribute and the importance of working in partnership with community members to bring about change.

In Chapter 6, material aspects of access were discussed along with social and political aspects. Examples were given of ways in which occupational therapists manage the material elements of a practice to facilitate access, such as adapting environments, changing location and finding new ways of utilising what is available.

Competences

As occupational therapy evolved into a cognisable set of practices, it became recognised as a profession with competences that could work with other healthcare practices. However, as described in Chapter 1, this primarily meant recognition by the powerful profession of medicine. This led to occupational therapy gaining more opportunities for healthcare practice but the profession lost most of its power to determine how and why its profession-specific competences could be applied. In Chapter 2, we explored how the managerialisation of healthcare services resulted in the reduction of professional roles to lists of tasks, allowing for more generic working. Aspects of care that used to be seen as the domain of particular professions can now be carried out by any person with the appropriate competences. This system is leading to a devaluing of professional skills and, over time, may bring about loss of profession-specific skills; as time for teaching and practising is taken up by generic working.

At the same time, there is pressure for occupational therapists, along with other health and social care professionals, to develop new, generic competences for working with diversity, intersectionality and complexity. The people who need our services most are those with multiple and complex problems, whose needs cannot be met by following a checklist of tasks but require high levels of professional reasoning. Competent professional reasoning is backed up by cultural sensitivity, resourcefulness, communication skills and pragmatism.

Several chapters in the book explore how the professional competence of occupational therapists is evidenced not by meeting people's needs but through assisting them to find ways of meeting their own needs. Most chapters explore how the needs expressed by individuals are the starting point for competent professional reasoning. However, when professionals are expected to work to the goals and values of the employing organisation, it becomes more difficult to put the needs of the client first.

Most chapters include examples of occupational therapists using different compe- tences to work with the macro- and micro-level issues that influence their practice. For example, Chapter 6 told the stories of an occupational therapist in Iceland, who found a way to set up a new service within the constraints of national political and economic policies, and an occupational therapist who was able to successfully transfer her mentoring role online when the COVID-19 pandemic put a stop to face-to-face meetings.

Meanings

Social practices, as we have seen throughout this book, arise from human experiences and are shaped by the long trajectory of development over time. In Chapter 1, we saw how occupational therapy developed out of the confluence of various social move- ments, demographic changes and historical events that occurred during the late 19th and early 20th centuries. These factors combined into teleoaffective structures that suggested a need for a particular set of practices to address social problems. Initially, this work was carried out by groups of women philanthropists, nurses, social workers and doctors in community settings, such as housing projects for the working poor.

From the meanings associated with this kind of work, which involved teaching skills and providing other forms of education and work opportunities, occupational therapy was developed. Common understandings of what was to be done, how it was to be done and why it should be done gave structure to an emerging social practice. The meaning of a practice is in its purpose, the ends it is intended to achieve and the beliefs and emotions associated with it. For example, the first occupational therapists saw their purpose being to engage people 'in some helpful and gratifying activity' (Meyer 1922/1977: 639) and 'to *obtain* performance wherever it had failed to come *sponta- neously* and thereby to serve the organism in the task of keeping itself in good form' (p. 641).

The meaning of occupational therapy has evolved over time and is not necessarily the same in different contexts. Nonetheless, occupational therapists around the world can agree on a common set of purposes and values that represent the profession. This book includes case studies from several continents and diverse settings that are all recognisable as occupational therapy practice. For example, in Chapter 8, three case studies demonstrate a continuous connection with the meaning of practice, despite changes in the material circumstances of the people the therapists were working with or in the structure of the services themselves. This connection allowed clients to ne- gotiate positive outcomes and continue to make progress, and occupational therapists to make continuing adjustments so as to maintain the value of their intervention with clients.

Structures

In Chapter 2, we saw how occupational therapists become subject to the teleoaffective structures of the health systems in which they work; such as management practices oriented to running an effective organisation and the availability of spaces in which to carry out occupational therapy. What the occupational therapist can do is prefigured by such factors as the design of the spaces of occupational therapy departments and the accounting practices that determine budgets and how services are costed.

Institutional structures might require various records to be kept, meetings to be attended and communications made or responded to, in addition to the delegation of parts of therapeutic practice. Both management practices and the design of services influence how authority, power and rules create social structures that impact on occupational therapy.

Structures can be conceptualised as having three qualities: jurisdictional, temporal and material-spatial (Blue and Spurling, 2017). Jurisdictional qualities are the authority that people have to carry out particular activities; temporal qualities are the ways that practices are organised in space and time, and material-spatial qualities determine the organisation of practices through the design or ordering of physical spaces and organisational structures. Examples were given in Chapters 3 and 6 of practices that were aligned with the negotiated needs of clients through structures that admitted the scope to answer these requirements.

From a practice theory perspective, social structures are created by the seemingly mundane practices that people engage in every day; these structures continue to exist only as long as daily practices keep being performed. This aspect of social practice theory allows us both to understand the social and historical context of the practices of everyday life and also to examine, at micro-level, the everyday practices that keep society functioning. An example given in Chapter 6 (Box 6.3) illustrated how what people in care eat for breakfast is determined by the choices offered through the catering structure. If the choice is limited, staff can easily assume that their clients have no other preferences because other possibilities have not been explored. This system reproduces monotony and restricts freedom of choice.

We have highlighted the four elements of occupational therapy as a social practice – materials, competences, meanings and structures – that have been explored in this book. The case study in Box 9.4 provides an illustration of how these elements interact in practice.

Box 9.4   Working independently

My title is Specialist Neurological Occupational Therapist, Elite Occupational Therapy Services Ltd. I have worked as an independent occupational therapist for the last eight years.

I have been an occupational therapist for 33 years, working in a range of posts and for statutory agencies, including the NHS and academia. Immediately before moving into independent practice, I worked in an NHS neuro-rehabilitation team. Despite enjoying the teamwork ethos, I realised that, in order to continue being an occupational therapist, I needed to leave the NHS. I considered the following options when making this decision.

In order to succeed within the NHS, in terms of career progression, an occupational therapist is required to fast-forward through their clinical grades and then cast aside that valuable experience and acquired skills to take up a management position. However, I believe that a management position within the NHS is a very limiting role since the NHS requires managers to administer policies and procedures. Despite much rhetoric regarding leadership, true leadership is not possible within this organisation. I value the critical and creative thinking skills developed during my years as an occupational therapist and my evidenced-based decision-making in rehabilitation. These would have to be put aside if I moved into a management position.

This led to me trade the safety and security of a job within a major statutory organisation for a future that I perceived to lack job security but that offered me opportunities to utilise the skills I valued. I saw that there was a demand for highly specialised occupational therapists offering rehabilitation, outside of statutory services, for people who had suffered a traumatic brain injury and who were pursuing a litigation claim.

The occupational therapy I provide is valued by the case managers who instruct me to work with their clients and by other professionals working in the client's treating team. Within this role, I can utilise my specialist skills fully. I am able to base my intervention plans on best evidence and consideration of my client's best interests, rather than on the service priorities of an organisation. I often describe being able to 'flex my muscles' within this role and 'practise proper occupational therapy'. My decisions regarding occupational therapy intervention need to be fully justified to the fee payer; however, there are no constraints on my decision-making. The freedom this provides is exhilarating but the responsibility is entirely mine!

I work within my clients' normal environments, including their homes, workplaces and social or leisure places: I avoid using clinical spaces, such as clinics, offices or gyms. I consider the environment to be a therapeutic tool. For example, a client may have the goal of being able to go out for a meal with their partner or family, which would involve being able to tolerate a noisy environment whilst following a conversation – a real divided attention challenge! With such a client, I might carry out a process training session in a café or restaurant, as part of a cognitive rehabilitation programme. Carrying out process training within that environment means that the client can directly transfer attentional skills to the real-life situation much more easily than if they practised them within a clinic or office setting.

I have enjoyed learning business-related skills. As an independent occupational therapist, I was required to learn how to set up the business of occupational therapy. I invoice the fee payer, sometimes an insurer or the person holding an interim funding payment for rehabilitation, at the end of each month for each client. Every time I do this, I feel a sense of pride in invoicing 'for the provision of occupational therapy services'. I am selling a product I can be proud of.

All of my income is derived from providing specialist occupational therapy services and, after my first year, I have been able to secure enough work and income to exceed my NHS salary. However, income can be sporadic. If I am on holiday, or take time off due to illness, I do not have any income. If I do not receive referrals, or perhaps the intervention for a client has to be paused or ceased due to a lack of funding in a case, then I do not receive an income. I therefore have to dedicate time to seeking work. This is through the development of a website, using social media and networking. This is all unbillable time and also carries costs. I contribute to a pension scheme and have to spend time on accounting so that all necessary taxes are paid.

Having worked within the NHS and now in the medico-legal sector has made me acutely aware of the lack of statutory services for people with acquired brain injuries. I therefore provide two hours a week pro bono to my local Headway branch. Headway is a national charity supporting people with brain injuries. There are many opportunities for voluntary provision of occupational therapy services within this sector and many independent occupational therapists provide pro bono hours but, interestingly, I am not aware of occupational therapists from the NHS undertaking this kind of voluntary work.

This case study shows the interaction of materials, competences, meanings and structures in the work of an independent occupational therapy practitioner.

Angela says that she misses some aspects of the materiality of working in the NHS, such as teamwork. However, in her current role, as an independent practitioner, she is able to utilise the materials available in the client's everyday environments to tailor interventions to their specific needs, rather than working within the environment of a hospital or clinic.

Angela observes that working independently allows her to use her full range of skills and expertise, which are valued by funders and clients. Her jobs within the NHS, where outcome goals tend to be defined by the organisation rather than the client, did not utilise all her competence or provide continuing opportunities for new learning.

Angela felt that, in her NHS role, her expertise was not sufficiently valued for her to progress up the career ladder as a practitioner. In order to reach a higher pay grade, she would have to change the meaning of her work and become a manager. Working independently, she was able to hold onto the meaning of her profession by continuing to enact a clinical role, without losing out financially. Indeed, she is so financially successful that she is able to offer pro bono specialist services to the local branch of a national charity.

Finally, working independently gives Angela the autonomy to develop a business structure that suits the needs of clients, funders and herself. This is in contrast to her work in the NHS, which tended to be structured to meet the needs of the employing organisation.

Summary and conclusion

This chapter began with a discussion of how the practices of occupational therapy are aligned both with medical goals and processes and also with social justice and reform. We have emphasised that occupation remains the basis of occupational therapy practice in the diverse contexts in which the profession has established that meaning. In the 21st century, faced with social and environmental issues that impact occupations and livelihoods around the world, occupational therapists are developing new theories and approaches that enable their services to remain socially relevant. In the last section of the chapter, the elements of occupational therapy as a social practice were summarised, with an illustrative example.

Throughout the book, we have explored various examples of practice, both from within mainstream health and social care services and in settings where structures are less well defined. Occupational therapy emerged as a profession just over a century ago and has subsequently developed into a global profession. Working with what people do, across different societies and contexts around the world, occupational therapists have had to continually adapt and innovate their practices, often using whatever resources can be found to support their work. They have also had to adapt their goals, methods and approaches to meet the needs of different communities and cultures and to fit within existing social structures.

During its more than 100 years of existence, the occupational therapy profession has aligned itself with medicine, in order to have its practices recognised and legitimated, but it has also formed its own organisations, including national colleges and associations; regional and continent-wide associations, and the international professional body, the World Federation of Occupational Therapists. Increasingly, the efficacy and cost-effectiveness of occupational therapy interventions are supported by a body of evidence, disseminated through the profession's international journals. The development of an underpinning theory of occupational science continues to expand and connect different strands of interest. Much of this flow of dissemination reflects the experiences of the Global North and the anglophone world but, increasingly, the voice of the majority world is influencing the shape and content of occupational therapy knowledge.

Occupation is the means by which people engage directly with the world, in all its complexity, and is therefore dynamic. Occupational therapy must reflect the increasing diversity and intersectionality in societies. Practitioners need to navigate practice environments that are characterised by complexity. They have to recognise and embrace new opportunities while recognising the values of interconnectedness that guarantee sustainability.

Throughout this book, we have argued that the current knowledge base and professional reasoning skills of practitioners are proving inadequate to explain and support occupational therapy practice in diverse settings. We suggest that practice theory might help the profession to develop new, effective, context-specific strategies that will assist practitioners in developing interventions and navigating structures outside mainstream health and social care services.

References

Bruggen, H. v., Craig, C., Kantartzis, S., Laliberte Rudman, D., Piskur, B., Pollard, N., Schiller S., and Simó, S. (2020) *Case studies for social transformation through occupation.* Vienna: ENOTHE Online at https://enothe.eu/wp-content/uploads/2020/06/ISTTON-booklet-final.pdf. Accessed May 2022.

Brymer, E., Freeman, E., and Richardson, M. (2019) One health: the well-being impacts of human-nature relationships. *Frontiers in Psychology*, 10: 1611.

Bukhave, E.B., and Creek, J. (2021) Occupation through a practice theory lens. *Journal of Occupational Science*, 28(1): 95–101.

Çaya, S. (2016) Cultural aspects of being poor. *Cross-Cultural Communication*, 12(2): 32–42.

Chadwick, D., Ågren, K.A., Caton, S., Chiner, E., Danker, J., Gómez-Puerta, M., Heitplatz, V., Johansson, S., Normand, C.L., Murphy, E., and Plichta, P. (2022) Digital inclusion and participation of people with intellectual disabilities during Covid-19: a rapid review and international bricolage. *Journal of Policy and Practice in Intellectual Disabilities*. 10.1111/jppi.12410

Chapparo, C., and Ranka, J. (1997) Towards a model of occupational performance: model development. *Occupational Performance Model (Australia): Monograph*, 1: 24–45. Online at https://citeseerx.ist.psu.edu/viewdoc/download?doi=10.1.1.503.4713andrep=rep1andtype=pdf. Accessed May 2022.

Chuwa, L.T. (2014) *African indigenous ethics in global bioethics: interpreting Ubuntu* (Vol. 1). New York: Springer.

Creek. J., and Cook, S. (2017) Learning from the margins: enabling effective occupational therapy. *British Journal of Occupational Therapy*, 80(7): 423–431. 10.1177/0308022617701490

Delhey, J., Schneickert, C., and Steckermeier, L.C. (2017) Sociocultural inequalities and status anxiety: redirecting the spirit level theory. *International Journal of Comparative Sociology*, 58(3): 215–240.

Drury, P., and Lazuardi, L. (2021) Telehealth and digital inclusion in Indonesia. Oxford: High-quality technical assistance for results (HEART). Online at https://www.heart-resources.org/wp-content/uploads/2022/01/Telehealth-and-Digital-Inclusion-in-Indonesia-Full-Report.pdf. Accessed May 2022.

Dunn, W., Brown, C., and McGuigan, A. (1994) The ecology of human performance: A framework for considering the effect of context. *The American Journal of Occupational Therapy*, 48(7): 595–607.

Dunn, W. (2017) The ecological model of occupation. In J. Hinijosa, P. Kramer, and C.B. Royeen (eds) *Perspectives on human occupation: theories underlying practice*. Philadelphia: FA Davis. 207–235

Fung, A. (2015) Putting the public back into governance: the challenges of citizen participation and its future. *Public Administration Review*, 75(4): 513–522.

Galvaan, R., and Peters, L. (2014) Occupation-based community development framework Online at https://vula.uct.ac.za/access/content/group/9c29ba04-b1ee-49b9-8c85-9a468b556ce2/OBCDF/index.html. Accessed May 2022.

Geilinger, N., Haefliger, S., von Krogh, G., and Rechsteiner, L. (2016) What makes a social practice? Being, knowing, doing and leading. *European Management Journal*, 34(4): 319–327.

Graham, R. (2017) *The lived experiences of food insecurity within the context of poverty in Hamilton, New Zealand*: a thesis presented in partial fulfilment of the requirements for the degree of Doctor of Philosophy in Psychology at Massey University, Albany, New Zealand. Doctoral dissertation, Massey University. Online at https://mro.massey.ac.nz/handle/10179/13001. Accessed May 2022.

Gramsci, A. (1971) *Selections from the prison notebooks*, edited and translated by Quintin Hoare and Geoffrey Nowell Smith. London: Lawrence and Wishart.

Greenhalgh, T., and Papoutsi, C. (2018) Studying complexity in health services research: desperately seeking an overdue paradigm shift. *BMC Medicine*, 16: 95. 10.1186/s12916-018-1089-4

Greer, B., Robotham, D., Simblett, S., Curtis, H., Griffiths, H., and Wykes, T. (2019). Digital exclusion among mental health service users: qualitative investigation. *Journal of Medical Internet Research*, 21(1): e11696.

Hitch, D., Pépin, G., and Stagnitti, K. (2014) In the footsteps of Wilcock, part one: the evolution of doing, being, becoming, and belonging. *Occupational Therapy in Health Care*, 28(3): 231–246. 10.3109/07380577.2014.898114

Hoel, V., Zweck, C.V., Ledgerd, R., and World Federation of Occupational Therapists (2021) The impact of COVID-19 for occupational therapy: findings and recommendations of a global survey. *World Federation of Occupational Therapists Bulletin*, 77(2): 1–8.

Hoofnagle, C., Kesari, A., and Perzanowski, A. (2019) The tethered economy. *George Washington Law Review*, 87(4): 783–874.

Hooper, B., and Wood, W. (2002) Pragmatism and structuralism in occupational therapy: the long conversation. *American Journal of Occupational Therapy*, 56(1): 40–50.

Ikiugu, M.N. (2008) *Occupational science in the service of Gaia*. Baltimore, MD: PublishAmerica.

Joubert, R. (2009) Are we the victims of our history? *South African Journal of Occupational Therapy*, 39(1): 1–1.

Lamb, A.J. (2017) Presidential address, 2017-Unlocking the potential of everyday opportunities. *The American Journal of Occupational Therapy*, 71: 6. 10.5014/ajot.2017.716001

Litchfield, I., Shukla, D., and Greenfield S. (2021) Impact of COVID-19 on the digital divide: a rapid review. *BMJ Open*, 11: e053440. 10.1136/bmjopen-2021-053440

Lopes, R.E., and Malfitano, A.P.S. (eds.) (2020) *Social Occupational Therapy*. Edinburgh: Elsevier

Lueddeke, G.R., Kaufman, G.E., Lindenmayer, J.M., and Stroud, C.M. (2017) "Preparing society to create the world we need through 'One health' education". *South Eastern European Journal of Public Health* (SEEJPH). 10.4119/seejph-1858

Lythreatis, S., Singh, S.K., and El-Kassar, A.N. (2021) The digital divide: a review and future research agenda. *Technological Forecasting and Social Change*, 175. 10.1016/j.techfore.2021.121359

Macdonald, E.M. (1961) The responsibility of exporting a profession—opening an occupational therapy training school in the argentine. *Occupational Therapy: the Official Journal of the Association of Occupational Therapists*, 24(6): 14–19.

McDonald, D.A. (2010) Ubuntu bashing: the marketisation of 'African values' in South Africa. *Review of African Political Economy*, 37(124): 139–152. 10.1080/03056244.2010.483902

Mattingly, C., and Fleming, M.H. (1994) *Clinical reasoning: Forms of inquiry in a therapeutic practice*. Philadelphia: FA Davis.

Meyer, A. (1922/1977) The philosophy of occupation therapy. *American Journal of Occupational Therapy*, 31(10): 639–642.

Monzeli, G.A., Morrison, R., and Lopes, R.E. (2019) Histories of occupational therapy in Latin America: the first decade of creation of the education programs. *Cadernos Brasileiros de Terapia Ocupacional*, 27: 235–250.

Mourão, I., Mouro, C.V., Brito, L.M., Costa, S.R., and Almeida, T.C. (2022) Impacts of therapeutic horticulture on happiness and loneliness in institutionalized clients with mental health conditions. *British Journal of Occupational Therapy*, 85(2): 111–119. 10.1177/0308022 6211008719

National Heath Service (2019) The NHS long term plan. Online at https://www.longtermplan. nhs.uk/publication/nhs-long-term-plan/. Accessed May 2022.

Nicolini, D. (2012). *Practice theory, work and organization: an introduction*. Oxford: Oxford University Press.

Ninnis, K., Van Den Berg, M., Lannin, N.A., George, S., and Laver, K. (2019) Information and communication technology use within occupational therapy home assessments: a scoping review. *British Journal of Occupational Therapy*, 82(3): 141–152.

Nobakht, Z., Rassafiani, M., Hosseini, S.A., and Ahmadi, M. (2017) Telehealth in occupational therapy: a scoping review. *International Journal of Therapy and Rehabilitation*, 24(12): 534–538.

Parkinson, S., Shenfield, M., Reece, K., and Fisher, J. (2011) Enhancing professional reasoning through the use of evidence-based assessments, robust case formulations and measurable goals. *British Journal of Occupational Therapy*, 74(3): 148–152.

Pentland, D. (2021) Is anything in life simple? Why we should think about complexity. *British Journal of Occupational Therapy*, 84(7): 397–399.

Pollard, N., Viana-Moldes, I., Fransen-Jaïbi, H., and Kantartzis, S., The ENOTHE (European Network of Occupational in Higher Education) citizenship project group (2020) Occupational therapy on the move: on contextualising citizenships and epistemicide. In: R. Lopes and A. Malfitano (eds.) *Social occupational therapy*. Edinburgh: Elsevier. 151–163

Public Health England (2020) Disparities in the risk and outcomes of covid-19. London: Public Health England. Online at https://assets.publishing.service.gov.uk/government/uploads/

system/uploads/attachment_data/file/908434/Disparities_in_the_risk_and_outcomes_of_
COVID_August_2020_update.pdf. Accessed May 2022.

Schatzki, T. (2010) Materiality and social life. *Nature and Culture*, 5(2): 123–149.

Shove, E., Pantzar, M., and Watson, M. (2012) *The dynamics of social practice: everyday life and how it changes*. London: Sage.

Thomas, J., Barraket, J., Wilson, C.K., Cook, K., Louie, Y.M., Holcombe-James, I., Ewing, S., and MacDonald, T. (2018) Measuring Australia's digital divide: the Australian digital inclusion index 2018, RMIT University, Melbourne, for Telstra Online at https://apo.org.au/sites/default/files/resource-files/2018-08/apo-nid184091_5.pdf. Accessed May 2022.

Townsend, E.A. (1993) Muriel driver memorial lecture: occupational therapy's social vision. *Canadian Journal of Occupational Therapy*, 60: 174–184. 10.1177/000841749306000403

Townsend, E.A. (1998) *Good intentions overruled: a critique of empowerment in the routine organization of mental health services*. Toronto: University of Toronto Press.

Townsend, E.A., and Marval, R. (2013) Can professionals actually enable occupational justice?/Profissionais podem realmente promover justiça Ocupacional?. *Cadernos de Terapia Ocupacional da UFSCar*, 21(2): 215.

United Nations (n.d.). *Transforming our world: the 2030 agenda for sustainable development*. Online at https://sdgs.un.org/2030agenda. Accessed May 2022.

van Breda, A.D. (2019) Developing the notion of Ubuntu as African theory for social work practice. *Social Work*, 55(4): 439–450.

Walton, E. (2018) Decolonising (through) inclusive education? *Educational Research for Social Change*, 7(SPE): 31–45. 10.17159/2221-4070/2018/v7i0a3

Weisz, G., Cambrosio, A., Keating, P., Knaapen, L., Schlich, T., and Tournay, V.J. (2007) The emergence of clinical practice guidelines. *The Milbank Quarterly*, 85(4): 691–727.

Wilcock, A.A. (1998) Reflections on doing, being and becoming. *Canadian Journal of Occupational Therapy*, 65(5): 248–256.

Wilcock, A.A. (2001a) *Occupation for health: a journey from self health to prescription. Vol. 2.* London: British Association and College of Occupational Therapists.

Wilcock, A.A. (2001b) *Occupation for health: a journey from self health to prescription. Vol. 1.* London: British Association and College of Occupational Therapists.

Wilkinson, R., and Pickett, K. (2010) *The spirit level. Why equality is better for everyone.* London: Penguin.

World Federation of Occupational Therapists, Shann, S., Ikiugu, M.N., Whittaker, B., Pollard, N., Kahlin, I., and Aoyama, M. (2018) Sustainability matters: guiding principles for sustainability in occupational therapy practice, education and scholarship. World Federation of Occupational Therapists. Online at http://www.wfot.org/ResourceCentre.aspx. Accessed May 2022.

Glossary

Access A way or means of approach or entrance' (Shorter Oxford English Dictionary 2002).

Activism Social practices based on collaboration and collectivity, where individuals can identify common problems, work out their own solutions and identify the changes needed (Holland and Lave 2019).

Affordances The relationships between the capabilities of the performer and the properties of resources in the environment, particularly material resources, that pre-figure how those resources might be used (Norman 2013).

Anthropogenic biomes Patterns of land use or human–environment interactions that result in altered ecosystems, such as dense urban settlements or agricultural croplands.

Authority A social position that confers power to enforce obedience or to influence action (Shorter Oxford English Dictionary 2002).

Communities of practice Processes of shared learning and knowledge exchange, either formal or informal, through which people can develop (Lave and Wenger 1991).

Competence One of Shove et al.'s three elements of practice; 'multiple forms of understanding and practical knowledgeability' (Shove et al. 2012: 23).

Concept A principle of classification that can guide in determining whether an entity belongs in a given class (Audi 1999).

Constellations of practice A number of interdependent practices that come together as a system; 'interconnected nets of materials and practices' (Morley 2017: 91).

Constraints Delimitations of the field of possibilities that exclude certain courses of action and leave others open.

Co-production In healthcare, the concept of co-production recognises that both service users and professionals can contribute to a shared understanding of service models and their delivery, and therefore both have a central role in the sharing of essential knowledge from their different perspectives and experiences (Realpe and Wallace 2010).

Cultural humility Openness to cultural diversity together with an acknowledgement that, in everyday interactions, no one can claim an objective or neutral position; everyone is involved in a subjective way.

Degrowth A policy of not increasing demands or seeking economic expansion.

Equality Ensuring each individual or group of people has access to the same quantity of resources or opportunities.

Equity Justice or fairness.

Hegemony Hegemony in this book refers to Gramsci's use of the term, which concerned not only the leading role of the dominant class in the economy but their ideological, moral and cultural dominance. This dominance is achieved by both the consent and the coercion of the social classes below the dominant class. For occupational therapists, who are part of the bourgeoisie or middle class through their professional position, this rests on representing some of the interests of the lower class (Gramsci 1971).

Macro-level An umbrella term for the culture and society that frame the structures of and relationships among social practices. A macro-level system is composed of cultural patterns, values, beliefs, political structures and economic arrangements.

Managerialism An ideology that promotes management as the optimal form of directing an organisation and the best way to ensure organisational success (Janse 2019).

Marginalisation A process of excluding categories of people from full participation in society on the basis of perceived difference, such as gender, race, social class, religion, sexual identity and physical disability (Duncan and Creek 2014: 461).

Materiality Relates to the ways in which objects influence practice. Materiality is a component of all social phenomena as part of the context in which practice takes place and the objects through which practice is enacted or developed.

Materials One of Shove et al.'s three elements of practice; 'objects, infrastructures, tools, hardware and the body itself' (Shove et al. 2012: 23); the physical components of a person's life that are essential to the performance of all activities.

Meaning One of Shove et al.'s three elements of practice; 'the social and symbolic significance of participation [in a practice] at any one moment' (Shove et al. 2012: 23).

Micro-level The smallest level of activity at which social practices can occur; the level of the everyday practices of individuals that keep society functioning.

Neoliberalism An approach to governing that favours free-market capitalism, small government, deregulation and reduction in government spending.

Nexus A connected group or series; a network (Shorter Oxford English Dictionary 2002). A nexus is a point at which things are connected through a combination of forces, social practices and materialities, possibly as a product of development over time.

One health model All health is regarded as part of a single, interactive system; from the health of individual creatures to that of the entire planet (Davis and Sharp 2020).

Place A space to which people ascribe particular meanings and values. A place acquires its placeness for people because of the practices associated with that place. Places are constituted and reconstituted by the practices performed within them (Pink 2012).

Power The relative capacity of people within a social system to direct or shape the actions of others.

Practice/social practice A routinised type of behaviour' (Reckwitz 2002: 250); the site where social life transpires (Schatzki 2002).

Practice-as-entity A temporally unfolding and spatially dispersed nexus of doings and sayings' (Schatzki 1996: 89); how a practice continues to exist for individual practitioners between their own moments of performance.

Practice-as-performance A practice in the moment of doing; a practice being performed by a practitioner.

Practice theory A collective term that subsumes a range of theories that take social practices as their main focus; a singular term to describe any one of the theories subsumed within the collective term and taking social practices as their central unit of analysis.

Pragmatism An American school of philosophy; 'the philosophy of "common sense", problem solving, activity, and adaptation, dimensions by which occupational therapists have traditionally bound themselves' (Breines 1986: 56).

Pre-figuration The way that possible courses of action are qualified by the arrangement of the social context, 'on such registers as easy and hard, obvious and obscure, tiresome and invigorating, short and long, and so on' (Schatzki 2010: 140).

Profession A particular type of social practice that is defined by certain, socially agreed features; a variable social position that depends significantly on social, economic and political contexts and on the existence of structures that support professional practice, including funding.

Professionalisation A process through which an occupational group moves incrementally from partial professionalisation towards full professional status (Hugman 1991).

Resource A stock or reserve that can be drawn on as needed (Shorter Oxford English Dictionary 2002).

Risk The possibility of danger (Lupton 1999).

Role reasoning A process of clarifying goals and responsibilities, setting boundaries, negotiating relationships and activities with others, and thinking strategically and ethically about what we do and don't do (Sherry and Oosthuizen 2017).

Rules Social mechanisms for directing people to perform specific actions in particular ways (Schatzki 2010).

Scholar A person who advances or refines the knowledge base of occupational therapy.

Scholarship The development and organisation of occupational therapy knowledge through study and research (Shorter Oxford English Dictionary 2002).

Social exclusion Denial of entry to, or participation in, the prevailing social system and its rights and privileges.

Social structures A structural ordering of ongoing social practices' (Dreier 2008: 22).

Social transformation Producing positive changes in society through activism.

Space

>   **Lived space** The relative position of things is determined by the perspective of the observer. Lived space is not merely physical but includes social, cultural, political, virtual, discursive, conceptual. social and other dimensions.

>   **Objective or mathematical space** A three-dimensional container, bounded by height, width and depth, in which no point is uniquely privileged over any other.

>   **Relational space** Experienced and used by each actor in relation to their past experience, current activities and concerns, personal characteristics and many other dynamics; existing in relation to other spaces.

Space-time Time and space become unified space-time through the interactions of human beings in time and space (May and Thrift 2001). Human experiences of time cannot be separated from human experiences of space because future-oriented human action structures how human beings organise the world spatially.

Spatiality The experiential quality of space; space as it is seen from the point-of-view of people doing things.

Teleoaffective structures Ends, projects, tasks, purposes, beliefs, emotions and moods' (Schatzki 1996: 89) that help to organise and order practices in time and space, and that guide and structure the range of possibilities for practice performances.

Teleoaffectivity The totality of teleological (goal-directed) and affective (value-related) orders associated with a practice.

Teleology Purposeful action.

Temporality Human understandings of past, present and future.

Theory A conceptual system or framework used to organise knowledge in order to understand or shape reality (Bryant et al. 2014).

Time A phenomenon that can be understood in many ways, including

> **Objective time** The flow and pace of events that can be measured by the ticking of a clock.
>
> **Subjective or lived time** A variable aspect of everyday life that is derived from subjective experiences of the social world.

References

Audi, R. (1999) *The Cambridge dictionary of philosophy,* 2nd ed. Cambridge: Cambridge University Press.

Breines, E. (1986) *Origins and adaptations: a philosophy of practice.* Lebanon, NJ: Geri-Rehab. Inc.

Bryant, W., Fieldhouse, J., and Bannigan, K. (2014) *Creek's occupational therapy and mental health,* 5th ed. Edinburgh: Churchill Livingstone Elsevier.

Davis, A., and Sharp, J. (2020) Rethinking one health: emergent human, animal and environmental assemblages. *Social Science and Medicine*, 258: 113093. 10.1016/j.socscimed.2020.113093

Dreier, O. (2008) *Psychotherapy in everyday life.* Cambridge: Cambridge University Press.

Duncan, M., and Creek, J. (2014) Working on the margins: occupational therapy and social inclusion. In: W. Bryant, J. Fieldhouse and K. Banningan (eds). *Creek's occupational therapy and mental health,* 5th ed. Edinburgh: Churchill Livingstone Elsevier. 457–473.

Gramsci, A. (1971) *Selections from the prison notebooks of Antonio Gramsci.* Translated by Q. Hoare and G. Nowell-Smith. London: Lawrence and Wishart.

Holland, D., and Lave, J. (2019) Social practice theory and the historical production of persons. In: *Cultural-historical approaches to studying learning and development.* Singapore: Springer. 235–248.

Hugman, R. (1991) *Power in caring professions.* Basingstoke: MacMillan.

Janse, B. (2019). Managerialism theory. Retrieved 18 March 2021 from toolshero: https://www.toolshero.com/management/managerialism-theory/

Lave, J., and Wenger, E. (1991) *Situated learning: legitimate peripheral participation.* Cambridge: Cambridge University Press.

Lupton, D. (1999) *Risk.* London: Routledge.

May, J., and Thrift, N. (2001) *Timespace: geographies of temporality*. London: Routledge. 10.4324/9780203360675

Morley, J. (2017) Technologies within and beyond practices. In: A. Hui, T. Schatzki and E. Shove (eds.) *The nexus of practices: connections, constellations, practitioners*. London: Routledge. 81–97.

Norman, D.A. (2013) *The design of everyday things, revised and expanded edition*. Cambridge, MA: MIT Press.

Pink, S. (2012) *Situating everyday life*. Los Angeles: Sage.

Realpe, A., and Wallace, L.M. (2010). *What is co-production?* London: The Health Foundation. Online at https://improve.bmj.com/sites/default/files/resources/what_is_co-production.pdf. Accessed May 2022.

Reckwitz, A. (2002) Towards a theory of social practices. *European Journal of Social Theory*, 5(2): 243–263.

Schatzki, T.R. (1996) *Social practices: a Wittgensteinian approach to human activity and the social*. New York: Cambridge University Press.

Schatzki, T.R. (2002) *The site of the social*. Pennsylvania: Pennsylvania University Press.

Schatzki, T.R. (2010) Materiality and social life. *Nature and Culture*, 5(2): 123–149.

Sherry, K., and Oosthuizen, A. (2017). Role reasoning in occupational therapy. Unpublished course notes, Department of Occupational Therapy, Faculty of Medicine, University of Antananarivo.

Shorter Oxford English Dictionary (2002) *Shorter Oxford English Dictionary on historical principles*, 5th edition. Oxford: Oxford University Press.

Shove, E., Pantzar, M., and Watson, M. (2012) *The dynamics of social practice: everyday life and how it changes*. Los Angeles: Sage.

Wenger, E. (1998) *Communities of practice: learning, meaning and identity*. Cambridge: Cambridge University Press.

Index

Note: Citations of tables are indicated in **bold**.

abandonment 153–4, 161
Abdu, L. 146
Aberdeen Royal Asylum 9
ableism 112
Aborigines of Australia 66; aboriginal
    children 44
Abramsky, S. 128
access 100–21; alternative understandings of
    101–4; barriers to 102, 105, 112–13; context
    100; definition 101, 183; enabling 113–15;
    everyday life 104–5; macro-level issues
    105–11; micro-level issues 111–18; naming
    and framing problems 114; not-for-profit
    services 110–11; OT and issues of 100–5;
    OT services 107–10; specialist mentoring
    115–18
accessibility issues 103–4, 108, 168
accident and emergency (A&E) 31
accommodation 122, 132
accountability 131–2
accountancy 117
accountants 2
accounting 145, 175, 177
acquiescence 87
activism: definition 91, 183; social 11, 91, 93,
    151, 165, 183, 185
adaptability 131, 139
Addams, J. 5, 7, 13
ADL interventions 108
Adolescent Socio-Educational Service
    Centre 160
adolescents 44, 139, 149, 153–4, 160–1
advocate role 53
aesthetics 6
affordance: definition 124, 183
Afghanistan 114
Afro-descendants 104
ageing: demographics of 85, 165
agencies 50, 129, 173, 176
agriculture 85–6, 88, 183
aides 9–10, 13–15

airports 126
alcohol 3, 114, 149, 155; addiction 149
Alers, V. 93
alertness 65, 117
Alexander, N. 103
Allen, M. 41
Amazon: workers 88, 101
American Journal of Occupational
    Therapy 165
ancestors: cultural beliefs 55–7
ancient history 167
Andreff, W. 82–3
Anglophone countries 9, 91, 93, 179
animals 91, 171
anthropogenic biomes 88; definition 183
anthropology 79, 94
anxiety 65, 108, 115
apartheid 65–6, 87
appointments: timing of 54, 136
appraisal systems 28, 35, 37
appropriate paper-based technology
    (APT) 137
appropriateness 116
apps 159–60
architects 11
Argentina 84, 171
armies 15
Arora, D. 54
Arrigoni, R. 153
art 6, 156
artefacts 123, 126, 137–8, 141, 144, 174
Artisans' and Labourers' Dwellings
    Improvement Act (1875) 4
artists 11
arts and craft movement 1, 5–7, 13;
    1880–1920 6
Asimov, I. 81
assertiveness 117, 133
assistive devices 52, 73; *see also* devices
Astley Ainsley Institution 78
asylums 8, 13, 15, 149

asylum-seekers 64
atomic clocks 42
Attention deficit hyperactivity disorder
  (ADHD) 115
Audi, R. 7, 92, 143, 183
audit 27, 32
austerity 29, 36
Australia 9, 66, 85, 105; digital inclusion 182;
  first nations people 44; government policy
  44; Occupational Performance Model
  (AOPM) 170; occupational therapy 141
autarchy 160
authority: definition 29–30, 183;
  managerialism and 29–30
autism 36–8, 112, 149
auto-immune disease 88
autotelic occupations 103

babies 34
Badcock, E. 100
Baggs, M. 112
baking 54
banking 82, 85, 109, 143
Bannigan, K. 92
Barker, R. 24
Barnes, C. 102
Barnett, H. 4–5, 13
Barnett, S. 4–5
Barr, L. 34
Barreiro, R. G. 151
Barros, F. B. M. 150
Barros, S. 149
Barton, G. 6, 8, 13
Basaglia, F. 149, 151, 163
bathing 54, 79–80, 127, 159
bathroom adaptations 70, 79
Beagan, B. L. 85, 87, 91
Beaulac, W. L. 84
bed-rest 57
beliefs 144
benefit systems: punitive 168
Benetton, M. J. 151–3, 155, 161, 163
Benner, A. D. 44
Bezuidenhout, M. 57
bias 79, 150
Bickel, L. 86
bicycles 146
Bigby, C. 105
biodiversity 88
biomedical practice 70, 91, 165–6, 170; OT as
  a 166–7
biomedicine 90, 93
bird flu 91
Birleson, A. 176
black population 93, 104, 148, 169
Black, J. 82
blacksmiths 143

Blackwell, E. 3
Blad, C. 82–3, 88
Bollnow, O. T. 45
Bolt, M. 90
bonding 136
Book of Thoughts 154
boredom 8
Borthwick, A. 78, 91
Boston School of Occupational Therapy 10
Bottinelli, M. M. 84, 90
Bourdieu, P. 67
bourgeoisie 184
Brasil 148–9
Brazil 147–52; background to 147–8; *favelas*
  94; healthcare in 148–50; history of OT in
  150–1; mental healthcare, development of
  148–50; social activism in OT 151–2;
  Unified Health System (SUS) 148
Brazilian Centre for Health Studies 150
Brazilian Institute of Geography and
  Statistics (IBGE) 147
Brazilian Journal of Occupational Therapy 158
bread-making 54, 127
breakfast 42, 105, 176
Breines, E. 7–8, 185
bricklayers 155
Briguet, A. P. 155
Brinkmann, K. 86
British Empire 3, 9, 14, 82
British Library 25
Brodsky, B. 113
Bronfenbrenner, U. 106
Bruder, J. 88
Bryant, W. 92, 186
Brymer, E. 171, 173
budgeting 87, 133, 135, 139, 167, 175
Bukhave, E. B. 100, 110, 166, 168, 170
Burke, J. P. 92
buses 20, 117

Cameroon 69
Canadian 3, 5–6, 8–11, 15–16, 21–2, 44, 66,
  77, 99, 121, 166, 182
Canadian Occupational Performance Model
  92, 97
Canadian Society of Occupational Therapists
  of Manitoba 8
cancer 107–8, 110–11
capitalism 6, 28, 82, 184
CAPSad 149, 155–7
CAPSij 149, 153–4
carbon storage 88
Cardinalli, I. 151–2
cashless society 109
Casson, E. 4, 10, 13, 78
catering 32, 145, 176
cattle 65, 88

cerebral palsy (CP) 52, 55, 69
Chadwick, E. 4, 169–70
change in occupational therapy 143–64;
   context 143; definition of 'change' 143–6;
   healthcare provision 146–7; macro-level
   influences 147–52; manner of occurrence
   143–6; micro-level influences 153–60;
   person-centred processes 153–5; process of
   155–8; technological innovation and
   158–60; *see also* Brazil
Chapman, G. E. 85, 87
Chapparo, C. 170
charities 4, 28, 114, 128, 135, 138–9, 178
Chicago School of Civics and Philanthropy
   7–8, 10
children: Aboriginal 44; Brazilian 149–57,
   160–1; cerebral palsy (CP), with 52, 54–7,
   69, 72–4; child-friendly spaces 128; child
   labour 12, 142; childhood 2, 52, 55, 146,
   157; disabled 53; games of 19; holiday play
   schemes 139; literacy 126; parental pressure
   and 127; play and safety 63; refugees 128,
   130; sensory integration problems 108;
   settlement house movement 5; social
   categorisation 146; special needs, with 135;
   street 133; women's rights and 2;
   see also youth
China 125
cholera 3
Christian socialism 167
church buildings 104, 122
Church of England 3–4
Chuwa, L. T. 172
cigarettes 18, 64, 103; *see also* smoking
circus 130–2, 134, 141, 156–7; arts 130;
   equipment 132; performance 130; practice
   134; research 130; skills 131
CircusAid 130–2, 136–7; case study 130–7;
   resources utilised by **132**
citizenship 85, 148–9, 153, 160
clapping games 19
clay modelling 157
cleaning 88–9, 102, 124, 145
clergy 4, 122
Clewes, J. 24
client-centred practice 56, 70, 108, 116
Clifford Lathrop, J. 7, 13
climate change 80, 85–6, 88–9, 96–7, 99;
   unequal impact of 86
clinical experience **11**
clinical reasoning 55, 153, 160, 181
clinical services 26–7, 31
Clouston, T. J. 50–1, 104
clowns 157
cocaine 153, 155
cognition 52; cognitive awareness 117;
   cognitive rehabilitation 177

Cold War 85
collaboration 49, 91, 132, 161, 167, 170,
   172, 183
collectivism 75
colonialism 80–2, 85, 88, 94; colonies 14, 78;
   colonisation 44, 82; development 81, 93;
   heritage 14; legacy of 81–2; origins 84;
   policies 83; rule 14; societies 91
combustion engine 143
comedy 157
commodities 81, 169
commodity 66, 81, 83, 87, 169; OT as a 83–4
communism 106
communities of practice: definition 183
community-based services 69, 136, 138–9, 173
community occupational therapy 147
community psychiatric nurse (CPN) 138
commuters 64
competence 166; cooking 144; definition 19,
   123, 144, 183; practice theory 19
computers 82, 109, 128, 146; literacy 133, 146
concept: definition 183
confidentiality 116
conflict of interest 31
constellations of practice 80–5; definition 18,
   81, 183
constraints: definition 124, 183
consumables 127; definition 126;
   resources 144
consumption patterns 81, 85, 88
cooking 124, 127, 136, 138, 144–5, 149, 174;
   competences 144; definition 144; elements
   as a practice 144; materials 144;
   meaning 144
Cooper, K. 146
cooperativeness 133
co-production: definition 183
coronavirus *see* COVID-19 pandemic
corruption 148
cosmetologists 110
cost-effectiveness 48, 179
counselling 115, 149
COVID-19 pandemic: Brazilian approach
   158; contamination 91; digital
   marginalisation 169; DOTM and 153; face-
   to-face meetings, impact on 175; home
   visitations 73; hospital cancellations 33–4;
   improvisation 171; lockdown policy 158;
   mental health services 159–60; poverty,
   effect on 104; social gatherings, restrictions
   on 113; social isolation 159
Cox, D. L. 78
craft skills 31, 138–9, 160; *see also* arts and
   crafts movement
cramped conditions 73
Crawford, M. 31, 35
creativity 133

credit cards 109
Creek, J. 1, 24, 41, 47, 66, 92, 100, 102, 110, 113, 122, 129, 134, 165–6, 168, 170–1, 184
Creighton, C. 15
crime: criminal activity 82; criminal law 82, 100; rates 3, 63
critical occupational therapy 151
croplands 88, 183
crops 86
Crouch, R. 93
crowded spaces 63
Cruz, D. M. 148, 150
crying 157
Csikszentmihalyi, M. 103
Cuevas, D. 89
cultivation 80, 88, 124
cultural anthropology 99
cultural beliefs 43, 57
cultural humility: definition 183
cultural studies 17
cultural theories 67
cultural values 54
Cunningham, M. 91
curative services 15, 148
Curran, T. 112
customary practices 56
customs 123
Cutchin, M. P. 67

dams 125
dancing 172
Darley, G. 3–6, 13
Datta, R. 85
Davis, A. 5, 91, 184
day hospital 111, 158–9, 162
day room 61
day services 159–60
day-to-day practices 33, 36, 39, 47–8, 53, 58
De Certeau, M. 146
deadlines 117
death 2, 9, 71, 86, 102, 169
decentralisation 148
degrowth: definition 183
deinstitutionalisation 149
Delhey, J. 169
democracy 28, 39, 94
democratisation 148, 150
demographics 90, 143, 165, 173, 175
demonstrations 109
Denmark 9, 108–9
dentists 27
deportation 64
depression 108, 114–15
deprivation 102, 114, 130
de-professionalisation 34–5, 39;
    see also managerialism
der Merwe, V. 78, 95

deregulation 28, 30, 184
desertification 86
detention 113
devices 52, 73, 112, 126–8, 169; definition 126
Dewey, J. 7, 67
diagnostic assessment 36–7
Dickie, V. 67
dictatorship 94, 148, 150–1
dieticians 138
digital marginalisation 169
digital world 168–70
digitalisation 108, 146, 170
dignity 5–6, 113, 154
Diop, S. 86
disability: activism 112; disabled people 100–4, 112–13, 138; groups 108; inclusion 141; issues 151; liaison 102; non-disabled people 103, 112; nursing 120–1; personhood and 112; perspectives 102–3; policies 119; rehabilitation and 120; research 119; rights campaigns 101
Disabled Facilities Grant panel 79–80
disabled student allowance (DSA) 115
disasters, natural 86, 89, 143
discharge 37, 48, 53, 121
discrimination 114, 148, 161
disease 3, 11, 15, 30, 32, 71, 82, 86, 88, 91, 113, 146, 150, 172–3
displacement 80, 85, 89, 111, 125
Dituri, D. R. 152, 155
doctors 2, 11, 15, 26–7, 61, 78, 90, 110–11, 145, 175
documentation processes 133
'doing-places': definition 124
domestic service 3
domestic skills 12–13
dompas (paperwork) 65
donations 132
donors 50
Dorset House School of Occupational Therapy 10, 84
drainage systems 3
Dreier, O. 33, 101, 108, 123, 126, 135
dressing 54
droughts 86
drugs 30, 103, 114, 153–8
Drummond, A. D. 148, 150
Drury, P. 169–70
Duncan, M. 102, 184
Dunn, W. 168, 170
Durán, M. G. 89
Dynamic Occupational Therapy Method (DOTM) 151–3, 158, 160
dyslexia 115

Early Childhood Intervention (ECI) 55
East Anglian Sanatorium 9

ecological model 106
ecology 88; of human performance 168, 170, 180
economics 28, 49, 90, 93, 122, 125, 174; definition 125
economists 82, 85, 125
ecosystems 85, 88, 183
education: compulsory schooling 55; educators, role of 52; vocational 11, 150
Edwards, A. 133
Edwards, B. 26–7, 133
efficiency 15, 27
egalitarianism 7
Einstein, A. 45
Eisenhardt, K. M. 34
Ekwan, F. 143
elderly population 52, 54, 57, 64, 70, 73, 109
electric appliances 127, 138, 145
electricity 126–7, 138, 145
electronic communication 147
electronic goods 127
electronic record-keeping 145–6
electrotherapy machines 70
El-Kassar, A. N. 169–70
emergency care 29, 31, 122, 158
emigration 86
emotions 18, 20, 43, 46–7, 134, 144, 152, 156, 175, 186; emotional support 159; emotional trauma 113
engineers 11
entrepreneurship 133
environmental issues: challenges 55; changes 88, 143; conditions 168; factors 91, 172; health 99; issues 178; threats 88
epidemics 83–5, 150; *see also* COVID-19 pandemic
epidemiology 150
epistemology 11, 151, 165
equality 115, 182–3; definition 183; unequal development opportunities 126; *see also* inequality; inequity
equity: definition 184
Escorel, S. 148
ethics 103, 153, 180
ethnic minority groups 108, 148, 169
eugenics 103
European Union (EU) 139
evidence-based approach 55, 177
exploitation 14, 83, 85, 103, 130, 148, 161
extractive trades 14
eye contact 153

Facebook 64
face-to-face meetings 24, 49, 116, 147, 158–9, 175
facial disfigurement 101

facilitators 52
factory work 6, 25, 88
fairness 87, 115, 167, 184
faith-based approaches 55; *see also* religion
family 29, 71, 73–4, 137, 155; decision-making 57
Fantinatti, E. N. 152
Farias, L. 91
farms 172
farriers 143
fatigue 108
Favill School of Occupational Therapy 10
feedback 35, 38, 75, 116, 136, 140
feeding 54, 73, 79, 102
fees 49, 69; fee-for-service 49
feminism 93
Ferguson, H. 146
Ferrari, S. M. L. 150, 158
fibromyalgia 118
field of practices 16
Fieldhouse, J. 92
fieldwork 15, 130, 135
Fiocruz 149
Fleming, M. H. 165
Flinders, M. 82
'following' procedure 33
food banks 87
football 63, 123–4
forensic mental health 35
for-profit organisations 29
fossil fuel 85
Foucault, M. 67
France 15
franchise, universal *see* voting rights
freedom: of choice 105, 176; of expression 118; of movement 130, 143; of patients 149
Freeman, E. 171, 173
free-market economy 28, 30, 184
Freire, G. 151
Freire, P. 114, 151
Freud, S. 151
fridges 127
Friedland, J. 3, 5–6, 8–13, 15–16
friendships 168
Fulton, M. B. 9–10, 15
Fundação CASA 153, 160n1
fundraising 78, 131
furniture 71, 73, 139
future-oriented approaches 20, 45, 56, 62, 136–7
futurians 81, 93

Galheigo, S. 84, 151
Galvaan, R. 67, 170
games 19–20, 123, 158
gang violence 63

gardening 172
gardens 4, 13, 85, 128
gas 127
gate-keeping measures 170
Geilinger, N. 170
gender 90, 102, 125, 146, 152, 184;
  see also sexual identity
geodesic domes 132
geography 45, 73, 147
geological changes 143
geopolitics 152, 170
Germany: language 17; migratory
  movement 148
Giaccardi, E. 132, 137–8
Giddens, A. 17
Gilfoyle, E. 167
Giraldo-Pedroza, A. 85, 89
global issues 93; economy 82–3, 85; health 87,
  163; inequality 170; social issues 80, 85, 94
global north 82, 86, 88, 91, 179
global south 84, 91, 93
global warming 85
goal-orientation 20, 134
Goffman, E. 87, 112
Gomez, M. T. 103
government: definition 29
GPs (General Practitioners) 36, 138–9
Graham, R. 168
Gramsci, A. 151, 166, 184, 186
grassy spaces 63, 65
Greece 130–2
greed 82
greenfield sites 65
Greenfield, S. 169
Greenhalgh, T. 172
Greenlees, J. 146
Greer, B. 170
Grenier, M. L. 90, 93
Griffiths, R. 27
Griffiths Report (1983) 27
Griscom, J. H. 4
gross motor function 55–6
Grossman, H. 138
Guardianship Council 154
Guillebaud Report (1956) 26
gyms 63, 177

Haiti 82
Hammell, K. W. 14, 90–1
handicrafts 6, 9, 110
happiness 6, 132
hardware 19, 123, 126, 174, 184
Hauck, N. T. 150
Hawking, S. W. 45
Haworth, N. A. 13
Headway 178

healthcare: funding, time use and 49–50;
  see also COVID-19 pandemic; National
  Health Service (NHS)
hegemony 91, 166, 184; definition 184
Henderson, D. 10, 13
Hickman, M. J. 82
Hill, O. 3–4, 6, 10, 12–13, 167
Hilton, T. 6
Hinchliffe, S. 91
Hirsch, E. G. 8
Hitch, D. 93, 167
Hobbs, A. T. 10
Hoel, V. 171
Hofstede, G. 56
Hoggett, P. 28, 30, 32
Holanda, S. B. de 151
holidays 114, 139, 177
Holland, D. 90–1, 183
homelessness 63–4, 87, 107, 122; digital
  solutions 109
Hoofnagle, C. 168, 170
Hooper, B. 165
Hopi culture 43
Hopkins, H. L. 8–9
horizontal axes 118
horticulture 172
hospitals: complex of practices, as a 145;
  hospital life 106–7
housing: adaptations 79; associations 4;
  estates 3, 15, 138–9; management 2–3;
  managers 3–4, 12–13; multi-occupancy 4;
  projects 175; reform 1, 3–4, 11–12, 16, 23;
  studies 23; UK and US reform (1848–1875)
  3–4; *see also* settlement house movement
Howard, G. P. E. 27
Hugman, R. 8, 50, 185
Hui, A. 18–19, 63, 124, 187
Hull House Settlement 5, 7
human resources (HR): CircusAid **132**;
  macro-level issues 129; micro-level issues
  136–7; occupational performance and 124;
  see also resources
humanism 67
humanitarianism 83–4, 130, 151, 159
humility 134, 183
Humphry, R. 67
hunger 44, 144, 148
hunter-gatherer cultures 66
hunting 44, 80
Huot, S. 67

ice caps 88
Iceland 110, 175
ID measures: thumbprints 57
ideology 25–6, 34, 39, 47, 83, 173, 184
idleness 8, 89

Ikiugu, M. N. 89, 171
Illinois State Board of Control 7
illiteracy 126
illness 1, 13, 33, 56, 101–2, 111, 113, 151, 166, 177; *see also* mental health
imaginary spaces 134
immigration 1, 5, 7, 13, 43, 65
impairment-focused approach 48
impairments 52, 102
Imperial Order of the Daughters of the Empire (IODE) 3
imperialism 14, 85
improvisation 34, 137, 171
independent working 176–8
India 9
individualism 57, 67
Indonesia 88, 130
industrialism 6; cities 3; development 85; districts 5; expansion 5
industrialisation 3, 5, 12, 82; cities 147; countries/nations 1, 12, 25, 86
inequality: resisting social 84–5; social structuring of 82–3; *see also* equality
inequity: health and 87–8
infants 55
infection 3, 34, 102, 146, 169
infrastructure 19, 123, 126–7, 129, 174, 184; arrangements 127; cooking 144; definition 126
ingenuity 129, 137–40
injury 32, 53, 56–7, 113, 177
innovation 56, 81, 145–6, 158, 162, 165, 171
in-patient care 32, 36, 111, 113
inspectorates 32
Institute of Physical Medicine and Rehabilitation 150
institutional settings: working in 70–2
Institutional Shelter Services for Children and Adolescents (SAICA) 161n2
insurance 28, 36, 49, 158, 165
intention: definition 116
interconnectedness of practice 106, 111, 179
interdependent practices 18, 61, 145, 160, 172, 183
interdisciplinary approaches 110, 149
intergenerational practice 93, 128
Intergovernmental Panel on Climate Change (IPCC) 85
intergovernmental relations 84
International Classification of Functioning, Health and Disability (ICF) 66
International Monetary Fund (IMF) 84
internet use 169
internships 15
interpersonal skills 140
intersectionality 174, 179
intuition 133

Inuit adolescents 44
Iraq 114
Ireland, Republic of 82
island nations 69, 86
Israel 9
Italy 148–9, 163
Iwarsson, S. 108

James, K. 113
James, W. 7–8, 10
Jamrozik, A. 101
Janse, B. 26, 184
Japan: migratory movement 148
Jeyasingham, D. 147
Johansson, K. 103
Jones, M. 80
Jones, R. 13
Josephsson, S. 67
Joubert, R. 78, 172
jurisdictional qualities: definition 106

Kant, I. 45
Kanyeredzi, A. 105
Kenny, K. 82
Kesari, A. 168, 170
kettles: electric 127, 138
Khalsa, S. 3, 21
Khoisan identity 66
Kidner, T. 9–10, 13
kidney disease 32
Kielhofner, G. 92
Kings Fund 26–7
Kingsley, F. 137
Kiribati, Republic of 86
kitchens 124, 127, 144
knife safety 144
Knight, D. 81
knitting 117
know-how 18, 123, 125, 144
knowledge 144; knowledgeability, practical 19
Kuijer, L. 132, 137–8
KwaZulu-Natal province 52

labourers 4, 62–3, 65
Lake, D. 7
Laliberte Rudman, D. 96
Lamb, A. 165, 167, 172
Lancet, The 158–9
landlords 128
landowners 30
languages 91, 93, 105, 120; verbal language 116
laptops 128, 146, 170
Lathrop, J. C. 7–8, 13
Latin America 82–5, 167
Lave, J. 80, 90–1

Lazuardi, L. 169–70
leadership 27, 37, 133, 176–7
Leary, A. 32
legislation 3, 108, 149
Levin, H. 1
Levitt, R. 27
liaison services 31–2, 102
Lidz, T. 10–11
Liehr, S. 86
lifestyle 88, 155; coaches 110
Lima, E. M. F. A. 151
Linebaugh, P. 81–2, 87
linguistics 43, 108
Litchfield, I. 169
literacy 126, 146
livelihoods 125, 178
livestock 172
Ljósid 110
loans 82
lobbying 3
local authorities 3–4, 36, 79–80, 103
local communities 61, 125, 135, 138
local government 37, 135
Local Government Association 37
local labour 82, 132
London School of Medicine 2
Lopes, R. E. 78, 84–5, 89, 94, 151, 167, 170
Lorenzo, T. 129
Loy, D. R. 43
Lueddeke, G. R. 171
Luhmann, N. 106–7
Lupton, D. 113
Lussi, I. A. O. 150
Luthuli, A. J. 87
luxury goods 127
Lythreatis, S. 169–70

Macdonald, E. M. 13
Macdonald, G. L. 10
Macdonald, M. 84, 171
Machado, C. V. 148
macro-level issues: access 105–11; change in
    OT 147–52; definition of 'macro level' 184;
    human resources 129; managerialism
    28–33; material resources 126–7; personal
    capabilities 125–6; resource allocation 125;
    resources 124–9; space-time 127–8
macro-systems: definition 105–6
Madagascar 53, 74; OT training 74–6
Madeley, J. 83
Maglio, J. 130
Magnusdóttir, E. 110
Mahoney, W. 78
Malfitano, A. P. S. 89, 94, 151, 167, 170
management: definition 25; scientific
    principles of 25–6

managerialisation 26–7, 38, 145, 174
managerialism 24–40, 51, 79, 184; authority
    and 29–30; definition of 25–8, 184; de-
    professionalisation 35; healthcare services,
    management of 30–3; ideology of 25–6, 34;
    impact on occupational therapists 36–8;
    macro-level issues of 28–33; management
    25–6; micro-level issues of 33–9;
    neoliberalism 28–9; occupational therapy
    and 24; performance monitoring 35; power
    and 29–30; prefiguration 33;
    proceduralisation 34; rules and 29–30;
    sanctions 35–6; UK healthcare case
    study 26–8
manufacturing 85, 89
Marcolino, T. Q. 143, 151–2, 155
marginalisation 61, 90, 104–5, 112, 168–9;
    definition 184; digital 169
marijuana 153, 155–7
Marmot, M. 87, 91
Marques, I. P. 148–50
marriage 2–4, 54
Married Women's Property Act (1870) 2
Martin, P. 78
Marval, R. 167
Marx, K. 151
massage therapy 2, 68–9, 110
Massey, D. 44
material resources **132**; definition 123; macro-
    level issues 126–7; micro-level issues 134–5;
    see also resources
materiality: definition 184
materials 166; cooking 144; definition 19,
    144, 184
material-spatial qualities: definition 107
matrix support 149
Matsukura, T. S. 149
Maximino, V. S. 152
Max-Neef, M. 82, 88–9
Maxwell, E. 32
McCallion, L. 115
McDonald, D. A. 173
McGuigan, A. 170
McIntyre, S. 55
McKenna, H. 49
McKinstry, C. 130
McLynn, F. 81–2
meaning 166; cooking 144; definition 18–19,
    144, 184
Mello, A. C. C. 143, 152, 155
Melo, D. O. C. V. 150
memory 157
MENCAP 102
Mendez, M. A. 10
Mensah, J. 86, 89
mental ability 133

mental activities 18
mental health: in Brazil 148–50; charities 28,
   138; conditions 52, 181; diagnosis 113;
   diseases 15; disorders 149; healthcare
   148–9, 154; hospitals and institutions 8, 13;
   illness 1, 13, 101, 113; liaison 31–2; needs
   36; problems 34, 138, 149; promotion
   138–40; services 140, 148–9, 180; settings
   40, 138–9; suffering 150; teams 147, 153–4;
   wards 35, 120; welfare 4; well-being 116
mental hygiene movement 8
mental space 135
mental states 32, 63, 154
mentoring: specialist 115–18
Mercer, T. 102
Merriman, P. 45–6
mestizo population 148
Meyer, A. 8–10, 13, 175
micro-level issues: access 111–18; change in
   OT 153–60; definition of 'micro-level' 184;
   human resources 136–7; managerialism
   33–9; material resources 134–5; personal
   capabilities 132–4; resources 129–37; space-
   time 135–6
middle-classes 3–4, 8, 12, 15, 78
migration 12, 82, 89, 148
military: coup 84; dictatorship 94, 148, 150–1;
   government 84; hospitals 13, 15
Minkov, M. 56
mobile phones 169
Model of Human Occupation (MOHO) 166
Momori, N. 85
money laundering 82
Montag, W. 81
Monteiro, P. 18
Monzeli, G. A. 78, 84–5, 167
moods 20, 46, 117, 134, 186
Moore, T. 122
Morley, J. 18, 183
Morris, W. 6, 85
Morrison, R. 78, 84–5, 167
mortality risks 169
Morton-Nance, S. 102
Mosey, A. C. 100
motherhood 34, 54, 56
motivation 144
motorists 29
Mourão, I. 172
multidisciplinary practice 27, 48–9, 52,
   91, 158
multi-generational households 74
multinational corporations (MNCs) 83, 148
Murthi, K. 91
muscles 69, 177
museum sites 159
music 147; festivals 63, 65
myths 83

Namibia 95
Nancarrow, S. 78, 91
nannies 62–5
National Autism Team 37
National Health Service (NHS): accessibility
   listings 103; contracts 139; *long term plan*
   (2019) 173; managerialism and 25–8, 36, 38,
   176; mental health trust 138; OT schools
   78; pay grades 36, 177–8; white papers
   27–8; *see also* COVID-19 pandemic
National Society for the Promotion of
   Occupational Therapy (NSPOT) 7–9, 15
National Trust 3
Nazism 103
necro-economics 81
neoliberalism 24, 66, 106, 159; definition 184;
   economics 28, 90, 93, 149; governments 28,
   30, 87; ideology 39, 83; managerialism and
   28–9; policy 173; values 33, 39
Netherlands 90
network-building 139
neurodevelopmental therapy (NDT) 52, 68
neurodivergence 115–16
neurological conditions 53, 55, 69, 176
neurosis 149
New Zealand 9, 86
nexus: definition 184
Ni, X. Y. 86
Nicenboim, I. 132, 137–8
Nicholls, D. A. 79, 90
Nicolini, D. 18, 20, 25, 29–30, 67, 106, 123,
   166–7
Nightingale wards 145
Ninnis, K. 169
Nobakht, Z. 169
Nobel Prize 125
non-governmental agencies 50
non-governmental organisations (NGOs)
   110, 131
non-human resources 123, 127–9, 137, 140
non-medical staff 27–8
Norman, D. A. 124, 183
Northern Ireland 114
not-for-profit services 110–11
Novak, I. 52, 56
nurses 12, 61, 71, 110, 138, 146, 175; nursing
   officers 26
nursing 2, 65, 120–1, 145; care 32; history 162;
   profession 26, 90; staff 34
nurturing skills 12
nutrition 126

O'Sullivan, E. N. M. 11
obedience 30–1, 183
obesity 88
Obregon, L. 82
occupational therapy (OT): alternative

perspectives 12–16; arts and craft movement 5–7; biomedical practice, as a 166–7; climate change 85–6; colonialism, legacy of 81–2; commodity, OT as a 83–4; community 147; complexity 171–3; constellation of practice 80–5; contexts 78–80, 165; current status of profession 89–94; curriculum for **10–11**, 15, 95, 172; day-to-day practices of 47–8; developmental needs 170–1; digital world 168–70; displacement 89; early development of 8–12; education 10–11; emerging practice 93–4; exclusion from services 107–8; global exportation of profession 84; global social issues 85–9; goals of 48, 165–82; housing reform 3–4; inequality, resisting social 84–5; inequality, social structuring of 82–3; inequity and health 87–8; issues for 90–2; jurisdiction of 107, 109, 111; origins of 1–8, 12–14; practice 9–10; pragmatism 7–8; principles and practice 117; professionalisation 8–9; resources for **123**; settlement house movement 4–5; social practice of 92–4; social reform and 167–8; structure of 14–16; sustainability 88–9; theorising 11–12; theory and practice 78–99; therapists as advocates 79–80; therapists, role of 46–51; twenty-first century issues 80–5, 168–73; values of 48; women's movement 1–3; *see also* practice theory; social practice
oil prices 89
Okuma, D. G. 151
oligarchs 82
oncologists 110
one health model 91; definition 184
Ontario Society of Occupational Therapy 8
ontology 17
Oosthuizen, A. 53, 61, 185
oppression: internalisation of 87, 104
orchards 172
Organisation for Economic Co-operation and Development (OECD) 126
origami 159
orphanages 153
orthopaedic medicine 9, 13, 15
Orton, Y. T. 78, 90–1
outpatient services 36, 53, 73, 110, 149
outreach clinics 52; space-time 72–3
outsiders 69–70, 134
ovens 54, 127
overcrowding 3, 73, 86, 130
oversight, state 26–7, 53, 148
Oxfam 81, 88, 104, 170

Pacific Island nations 86
painting 88, 156–7

palliative care 108
pandemic *see* COVID-19 pandemic
Pantzar, M. 43, 46, 54, 64, 66, 122–3, 135, 166–7, 171
paperwork 65, 71
Papoutsi, C. 172
parameters: definition 116
parent facilitators 52, 57
Parkinson, S. 166
parks 88, 128
parole 113
Pastore, M. N. 151
Paterson, C. F. 2, 5–10, 12–13, 15
pathology 11
patriarchal structures 78, 90
Paulo Delgado Law 149
Peabody Trust 4
pedagogy 74–5, 151
PEG (percutaneous endoscopic gastronomy) 79
pensions 57–8; payments 57; rights 51; schemes 177
Pentland, D. 90, 172
Pépin, G. 93, 167
performance monitoring: managerialism and 35
Pernambucano, U. 150
Perón, J. 84
Perryman-Fox, M. 78
personal capabilities **132**; macro-level issues 125–6; micro-level issues 132–4; *see also* resources
person-centred approach 110, 153–5
Person-Environment-Occupation (PEO) model 66
personhood: disability and 112
Perzanowski, A. 168, 170
pests 82, 89
Peters, C. 78
Peters, L. 170
pharmacies 154
Philadelphia School 10
philanthropists 175; organisations 3–5
Philip, R. W. 13
philosophers 8, 10, 31, 67, 143, 166; accounts 59; discourses 1; movements 7; of occupation 181; of practice 21, 186; of pragmatism 7, 11
Phipps Psychiatric Clinic 8–9
physiological processes 54
physiotherapists 61, 68–9, 71, 110, 161
physiotherapy 68–9, 79, 85, 145
Pickett, K. 168
Pierce, C. S. 7
Pink, S. 64, 104, 184
place: definition 184
planetary health 85, 88, 173

plants 86, 171
plate-spinning 134
playgrounds 13, 63
pleasure 103, 117, 136, 155–7
pneumonia 48
polio 85
poliomyelitis epidemic 83–4, 150, 161
politics 68, 100, 122, 125, 140, 174; definition 125; political liberties 124–5
Pollard, N. 78–9, 143, 165, 173
populism 84, 143
porters 61
Portugal 148, 161
post-colonialism 66, 85
post-traumatic stress disorder (PTSD) 114
poverty 3–6, 54, 57–8, 73, 87–9, 94, 104, 111, 114, 128, 151, 166–8; impoverished areas 5, 13, 86, 129, 170
power: definition 29, 125, 184; managerialism and 29–30
practice: definition 184
practice-as-activity 18
practice-as-entity 17, 19, 93, 144–5, 160, 184; definition 184; practice theory 19
practice-as-occupation 18
practice-as-performance 17, 19, 145, 166, 185; definition 185; practice theory 19
practice theory 16–20; competence 19; conceptualising a practice 17–18; definition 185; elements of practice 18–19; main features of 17–20; materials 19; meaning 18–19; practice-as-entity 19; practice-as-performance 19; teleoaffective structures 20; *see also* social practice
pragmatism 1, 7–8, 10–11, 13, 23, 47, 174; definition 185
praktik (routinised behaviour) 17, 91
praxis: definition 17
prefiguration 33; *see also* managerialism
pre-figuration: definition 185
presidential addresses 165, 167
pressure sores 48
principles: basing practice on 117; definition 116
prison sentences 30, 160
prisoner rights 113
privacy 116, 159
private enterprise ventures 81
privatisation 82
pro bono hours 178
problem-solving 80, 130–1, 134
proceduralisation 34, 39; *see also* managerialism
Prodinger, B. 105
productivity 27, 31, 38

profession: definition 185; features 50
professionalisation 8–9, 24, 185; definition 185
professionalism 35
property 1–2, 4, 30, 65, 82, 86, 128
psychiatric care 149; conditions 154, 150; beds 149; clinics 8–10, 15; healthcare 11; hospitals 9, 149, 172; in-patients 113; medication 155; nurses 138; patients 10; reform 149; services 121, 153; symptoms 155, 157; units 120
psychiatrists 9, 150
psychiatry 9–11, 13, 69
psychoactive substances 149–50, 153, 157
psychoanalysis 151
psychological distress 153, 158
psychological medicine 22, 166
psychologists 11, 110
psychology 94
psychosis 149
psychosocial care 44, 120, 149, 153, 155, 161, 163
Psychosocial Care Centre for Alcohol and Other Drugs (CAPSad) 155
Psychosocial Care Network National Policy (RAPS) 149
psychosocial rehabilitation 149, 153, 163
psychotherapy 115, 149, 155
psychotic breakdown 153
public buildings 126
public demonstrations 109
public distrust 82
Public Health England 37, 169, 181
Public Health Act (1875) 3
public healthcare 110
public housing 128
public institutions 88
public law 160
public policies 98, 148
public sector 49
public services 28, 83
public spaces 61, 76, 128
public transport 63, 65
public utilities 82, 101
publishing 81
Purcell-Khodr, G. C. 44
'purposes' 144

qualifications 2, 78, 94, 101, 134
qualities: of connective tissue 76, 106, 119, 161; control 32; jurisdictional 106, 108, 110–11, 176; materials 83
quality: of care 27, 29, 31, 102; of life 5, 70, 119; of practice 26; of service 29, 148; of space 62, 186; technical assistance 180
quilting, patchwork 19

race 89–90, 102, 152, 184; spatial policies 65
racism 90
radicalism 148
radio 147, 159
radiographers 61
rail networks 126
rain 73, 86
rainforests 88
Ramugondo, E. 90–1
Ranka, J. 170
rapport-building 38
Rauch, T. 78
raw materials 14, 82
Realpe, A. 183
Reckwitz, A. 17–18, 67, 123, 184
Recommended Minimum Standards for the
    Education of Occupational Therapists 10
record-keeping 145–7
recreation 4–5
Red Cross Cottages 4
Red Cross Hall 4
Rediker, M. 81–2, 87
reductionism 48, 171
redundancy 36
Reed, K. L. 8, 10
Reeves, S. 35
referrals 36, 106, 110–11, 138–9, 177;
    questions 53
reflection, critical 75, 155
reforestation 88
refugees 65, 89, 97, 107, 128, 130; camps 70,
    111, 122, 128, 130–5, 140, 173; children 60;
    crises 86, 130; services 128; settlement 61;
    staff training 128; status 86
regionalisation 148
Regnard, C. 102
rehabilitation: centres 15, 110; practices 65;
    process 110; programme 177; services 71,
    90, 110, 150; teams 52, 72–3, 176; units 53;
    workshops 9, 13
Reid, H. 90
Reis, S. C. C. A. G. 94
relational agency: definition 133
relational space: definition 185
relativity, theory of 45
relaxation 19, 110
religion 14, 102, 104, 150, 184; God, role of
    55, 57; religious services 104
rent bills 3–5, 13, 31, 87, 128, 169
rental properties 128
Representation of the People Act (1918) 2
reservoirs 127
residential address 109
residential area 65
residential home 105
resource: definition 185; 'person' 52
resourcefulness 122, 135, 137–40, 174;

definition of 137–8, 140–1; OT in primary
    care 138–40; *see also* resources
resources 61, 122–42; adaptation and 131–2;
    CircusAid case study 130–7; context 122;
    definition of 122–4; identifying 130–1;
    macro-level issues 124–9; maximising
    131–2; micro-level issues 129–37; under-
    resourcing 29, 140; utilising 131; volunteers
    131; *see also* human resources; material
    resources; personal capabilities;
    resourcefulness; space-time
retail workers 169
rhetoric 82, 87, 176
Richards, G. 25, 85
Richardson, M. 171, 173
risk: definition 113, 185; taking 130, 134
Rivett, G. 26
role reasoning: definition 185
role-play 117
Røpke, I. 125
Rose, N. 26, 28
Rosenbaum, P. 55
rotas, staff 146
Rowland, H. 4
Rudman, D. 67, 91
rules: definition 29, 185
Ruskin, J. 6, 13
Russia: Ukraine, invasion of (2022) 143
Ryan, L. 82

Salles, M. M. 149
Salmon Report (1966) 26
Saloojee, G. 57
sanatoriums 9, 13, 15
sanctions 34–6, 39; managerialism and 35–6
Sanderson, S. N. 8, 10
sanitation 3–4
Sawyer, A. 101
Schafer, T. 102
Schatzki, T. R. 14, 16–20, 29, 33, 43, 45–7, 51,
    56, 62, 106–7, 125, 134–5, 137, 174, 184–6
schizophrenia 151
Schneickert, C. 169
scholar: definition 92, 185
scholarship: definition 92, 185
Schön, D. 8
School of Rehabilitation of the Brazilian
    Beneficent Association for
    Rehabilitation 150
Schwarz, L. M. 148
scorecards 37
Scotland 9–10, 15
Scottish Association of Occupational
    Therapy 9
Sedlačko, M. 16
self-harm 113
self-referrals 36

Sen, A. 124–5
Sennett, R. 6
sensory activity 79, 108
sensory-perceptual development 55
Serapioni, M. 149
Serrett, K. D. 11
settlement house movement (1884) 4–5, 13; *see also* housing
sewage 3, 89
sewing 19
sex 2, 103
sexual identity 102, 184; *see also* gender
Seyfang, G. 85
Shakespeare, T. 102
shame 87, 133
Shannon, P. D. 11
Sharp, J. 91, 184
Shefner, J. 82–3, 88
shelters 154, 161
Sherry, K. 41, 44, 53, 61, 185
shopping online 169
Shove, E. 18–20, 42–3, 46, 54, 64, 66, 92, 122–3, 126, 128, 135, 144, 166–7, 171, 174, 184
Shukla, D. 169
Shuma, B. E. 138
sickness 30, 37
Silberman, S. 103
SilentMiaow 112
Silva, C. R. 151
Silva, G. A. E. 148
Silveira, N. da 78, 150
Singh, S. K. 169–70
situational analysis 53
Sivasundaram, S. 14
skills 144
Slagle, E. C. 8–10, 13, 78, 167
Slater, T. 87
slavery 81, 87, 148
slums 3–4, 129
smoking 17, 64; *see also* cigarettes
snobbery 87
Soares, L. B. T. 150
soccer; *see also* football 20
social activism: Brazil 151–2
social consciousness 101, 112
social exclusion: definition 105, 185
social occupational therapy 94, 151
social practice: competences 174; definition 16–17, 184; materials 173–4; meanings 175; OT as a 165–8, 173–8; structures 175–8; theories of 16–20; *see also* practice theory
social reform: OT and 167–8
social structures: definition 185
social transformation: definition 91, 185
social workers 11–13, 78, 146, 150, 154, 175
socialisation 130, 136

socialism 6, 167
socio-cultural issues 64, 106, 168
socio-economics: developments 2, 57, 65, 76, 126, 143; factors 83, 91, 94, 170
socio-educational measures 160
socio-emotional development 55, 66
sociology 17, 66, 94, 104
socio-temporal ordering of practices 106, 111
software 168, 170
soldiers 9–10, 13, 15, 114
songs 159
Soto-Navarro, C. 88
South Africa 9, 42, 52, 57, 59–60, 65–8, 69, 76, 95–6, 172, 181
South America 84, 147–8, 167
South-East Asia 82
Southerton, D. 42
soya 88
space: context 66; environment 66; lived 62–4, 185; mathematical/objective concepts of 44–5, 62–4, 185; places for action 66; relational 63; relative 44; setting 66; spatiality, definition of 62, 186
space-time 42–6, 61–77; alternative spaces 73–4; battle of the chair 71–2; CircusAid **132**; concept of 61–2, 123; CP outreach clinics 72–3; cultural understandings 43–4; definitions 44–6, 62–4, 186; institutional settings, working in 70–2; lived time 42; macro-level issues 127–8; massage 68–9; micro-level issues 135–6; objective space 44; occupational science literature 66–70; OT literature 66–70; OT practice 68–70; OT training in Madagascar 74–6; place and space 64–5; practice, nexuses of 65–6; practice spaces, reconsidering 72–4; relative space 44; shaping spaces to enable practice 74–6; temporality and 42–6; *see also* resources; time/temporality
speech communication 147
Spiess, A. A. F. 90
spinal injuries 57
sponsorship deals 88
sports 20, 30, 88
Spurling, N. 61, 106–7, 145–6, 176
Stagnitti, K. 93, 167
Ståhl, A. 108
stamina 118
standardisation 75, 166–7; standardised procedures 31, 36
Stanley, B. 113
Starling, H. M. 148
Starr, E. G. 5, 7, 13
statistics 32, 37–8, 147
Statute of the Child and Adolescent (ECA) 154, 160–1
Steckermeier, L. C. 169

Stein, W. 113
Stephenson, J. 102
stereotypes 42
Stewart, S. 89
Stiglitz, J. 28
stigma 149, 151
stress 29, 114, 131, 136
subjectivity 45, 152
sub-Saharan Africa 172
suffrage 5; *see also* voting rights
suicide 44, 113, 154
Summerfield-Mann, L. 35
supervisors 52
surgeons, army 10, 15
surgery 53, 145, 159
surveillance 146
sustainability 24, 80, 85, 88–9, 136, 171, 179
Sweden 9, 109
Switzerland: migratory movement 148
system-centred approach 108
systemic structures 17

Tan, J. 44
Tansey, R. 29
task competence: without professional
    judgement 32
taxation 28, 82, 177
taxi drivers 53
Taylor, F. W. 25
Taylor, G. 7
tea breaks 47, 61, 70, 81, 139
teamwork 49, 133, 139, 176, 178; team
    members, abilities and needs of 133
Tebbit, C. 10
technological innovation: change in OT
    158–60
Tedesco, S. 152
teenagers 153–4, 160
teeth-brushing 75
Teitiota, I. 86
telehealth practices 158–60, 169
teleoaffective structures 17, 20, 33, 43, 47, 56,
    84, 175; definition 186
teleoaffectivities 24, 31, 46, 49, 51, 63; time/
    temporality 46–7
teleoaffectivity 20, 47, 50, 186; definition
    46–7, 186
teleological orders 40, 47, 56, 186
teleology 62, 106, 186; definition 186
temporal considerations 118
temporal qualities 106; definition 106
temporality: definition 186; *see also* time/
    temporality
tenants 3–4, 13, 128
Tenement House Act (1867) 4
tents 130
Tharoor, S. 14, 82–3, 88

theatre 149, 157
theft 30
theory: definition 92, 186
theory: of technique 151–2
Thew, M. 93
Thibeault, R. 72
Thomas, J. 169–70
Thornton, J. 102
thrombosis 145
time/temporality 41–60; clocks 42, 44, 49, 63,
    65, 186; context 41–2; cultural
    understandings of 43–4; definition of 42–3;
    experiential temporality 45; goals and
    decisions 56–8; life stage considerations
    55–6; lived time and OT practice 42, 54–5;
    management 49–50; objective time,
    definition of 42, 186; in OT practice 51–8;
    past, present and future 55–6; profession,
    features of a 50–1; role reasoning 53;
    service users, temporal realities of 54–5;
    space and 42–6; spending 49–50; subjective/
    lived, definition of 186; teleoaffectivities
    46–7; therapists, role of 46–51; time banks
    85; time zones 124, 127; time use, decisions
    on 52–3; *see also* space-time
Titchkosky, T. 66, 103–4
toileting 57; public toilets 101
Tomlinson, M. 42
Townsend, E. A. 167
Toynbee Hall 4–6, 23
Trade Union Congress (TUC) 101
training: child refugees 128; trainers, role
    of 52
transactional perspectives 67, 76–7
transportation 132, 154
trauma 11, 113, 130–2, 136
triadic relationships 152–3, 155–6, 158
Trimboli, C. 46
trousers 105
trust-building 136
Tuan, Y. 43, 64
tuberculosis (TB) 9, 13
tutors 110
Twinley, R. 90
Tyler, I. 87
typhoid 3

Ubuntu 172–3
Uganda 128
Ukraine: Russian invasion of (2022) 143
under-employment 101
undergraduate programmes 52, 150
under-representation 165
unemployment 65, 89, 114
UNICEF 55, 126, 128
Union of Physically Impaired Against
    Segregation (UPIAS) 102

United Kingdom (UK): army veterans 114; charities 128; exporting OT 78, 84; health and social care policy 90; housing reform (1848–1875) 3–4; imperialism and 14; managerialism 25–7, 34; professionalisation 8–9; training courses 10–11; women's rights (1800–1928) 2, 12; *see also* British Empire; colonialism; National Health Service (NHS)

United Nations (UN): development goals (2030) 171; Development Programme (UNDP) 148; homelessness 87; International Movement for Rehabilitation 150

United States (US): army 10, 15; Civil War 7; exporting OT 78, 84; health insurance 36; housing reform (1848–1875) 3–4; imperialism and 14; management 25; mental hygiene movement 8; older population and job security 88; OT schools 10; professional bodies and practice 7–10; reconstruction aides 9; settlement house movement 5–7; training courses 10–11; White House 101; women's rights 3, 12; World War I 15

universities 2, 5, 15, 78, 151

urbanisation 88; urban poverty 1, 3; urban settlements 88, 183

utensils 126, 144, 174

utility bills 87

utopian perspectives 85

van Breda, A. D. 172

van Bruggen, H. 168

Van Wyk, B. 66

Varoufakis, Y. 82, 99

veganism 145

Venezuela 89

ventilation 4

vertical axis 118

veterans 114

Victorian era 6

video clips 159

violence 63, 86–7, 111, 153, 161

virtual communication 159

virtual reality 32

virtual spaces 89, 124

vocational education 11, 150

voluntary hospitals 78

voluntary placement 53

voluntary provision 178

voluntary work 178

volunteers 4, 130–2, 136; resources 131

von Hoffman, A. 3–4

voting rights 2

vulnerability 138, 153, 167–8

Vygotsky, L. 18

wages 2, 88, 126, 128

waiting areas 73, 153

waiting times 37–8, 54

Wakefield-Rann, R. 88

Walder, K. 90

Walker, A. 85

Walker, G. 63, 124

Walker, J. 9, 13

Walton, E. 173

war 1, 9, 15, 63, 65, 129

wards 9, 13, 26, 35–6, 57, 65, 70–1, 73, 111, 120; aides 13; managers 26; occupations 9; patients 73; rounds 70; sisters 26; staff 71

water: access to/supply 3, 72–3, 86, 89, 126–7, 138, 144; as a sensory activity 79

Watson, M. 29, 43, 46, 54, 64, 66, 122–3, 125–6, 135, 166–7, 171

wealth 6, 14, 26, 81–2, 87, 125, 128

Weisz, G. 166

Welch, M. 101

welfare 4–5, 73, 88; history 7, 23; institutions 82; measures 166; programmes 5; provision 28

well-being 4, 38, 58, 105, 116, 125, 130, 137, 141, 152, 170, 179

Wenger, E. 80–1

West, W. 167

western cultures 56–7; democracies 28, 39; economics 83–4; society 57, 166; values 44; worldview 56

wheelchairs 72, 101, 115

Whipps, J. 7

Whitcombe, S. W. 50–1

white papers 27–8; *Agenda for Change* (1999) 27–8; *Working for Patients* (1989) 27

white population 65, 84, 148

White, T. 91

Whitfield, D. 27

Whybrow, S. 100

wi-fi hotspots 147

Wilcock, A. A. 1, 4–5, 8–9, 12, 47, 78, 84, 92–3, 167, 171–2

wilderness 88

Wilkinson, R. 168

Wilterdink, N. 100

Wiradjuri people 44, 85

Wolf, M. 88

women: African communities (*makhoti*) 54; chaperonage 2; craft groups 138–9; domestic skills 12; emancipation of 83; emotional resilience 138; rights of 2, 6–7, 11; suffrage 5; UK rights (1800–1928) 2; unmarried 3, 50; women's movement 1–3; *see also* children; feminism; gender

Women's University Settlement 4–5
Wood, W. 165
workhouses 13
working-class population 13
workshops 9, 13, 15, 81
World Federation of Occupational Therapists
   (WFOT) 9–10, 22–3, 46, 60, 121, 182
World Health Organization (WHO) 66, 84,
   86, 158
World Meteorological Organization
   (WMO) 86
World War I (WWI) 9, 11, 15
Wrenn, M. V. 83

Wright, T. 101
Wylde, E. 24, 36

X-rays 57, 70

Yalmambirra 44
yoga 117
youth 89, 149, 153; *see also* children

Zaidi, A. 85
Zambia 144
zero-hours contracts 88
Zulu 54, 172

Printed in the United States
by Baker & Taylor Publisher Services

Printed in the United States
by Baker & Taylor Publisher Services